Praise for

Living Bliss

*"Dr. C. Norman Shealy, a remarkable and highly developed soul, has written a very thoughtful, thought provoking, and entertaining book, **Living Bliss.** It is a healing gift of monumental proportion that lovingly adds to the almost unaccountable contributions he has made to both orthodox complementary and holistic alternative medicine in our space/time world.*

"This book is a kind of crowning capstone that Dr. Shealy has given to the great pyramid of his prolific number of individual contributions and gifted to humanity in this remarkable current lifetime.

"Just as the human acupuncture meridian system of our first subtle body is the template that energizes and nourishes all aspects of our course electric physical body, in Dr. Shealy's new book the five sacred rings of specific meridian-point stimulation via the five specific bliss oils bring healing to a plethora of significant human ailments! Bravo, Norm, bravo!"

— **William A. Tiller, Ph.D.**, professor emeritus of materials science at Stanford University and author of three major books on the power of conscious intentions

*"For four decades Dr. Norm Shealy has taught people how to live not only long but also well. In **Living Bliss**, he breaks down the walls between the physical, emotional, and spiritual aspects of our being. This extraordinary pioneer of healing continues to show us that the medicine of the future is available now."*

— **Larry Dossey, M.D.**, author of
The Power of Premonitions and *Reinventing Medicine*

*"**Living Bliss** is an extraordinary book from a great man. I highly recommend it and its life-changing information."*
— **Christiane Northrup, M.D.**, ob-gyn, physician, and author of the *New York Times* bestsellers *Women's Bodies, Women's Wisdom* and *The Wisdom of Menopause*

*"Dr. Norm Shealy has been a pioneer in the field of health and wellness for decades, and he shows no signs of slowing down! I read **Living Bliss** cover to cover and immediately implemented some potent suggestions into my life. I highly recommend you read this book today!"*
— **Nick Ortner**, *New York Times* best-selling author of *The Tapping Solution*

*"If you are searching for physical, psychological, and spiritual well-being, then Dr. Norm Shealy's new book **Living Bliss** is indispensable. A word of caution, however: Dr. Shealy takes no prisoners and pulls no punches. He is meticulous in his evaluations, scrupulous in his scientific conclusions, and magical in his formulations—but uncompromising in his discussions of humanitarian obligations. This is not a book for the sanctimonious, the maudlin, or the fundamentalist. I found his no-nonsense delivery and straightforward honesty refreshing, and I know you will as well! I strongly urge you to read this book!"*
— **Eldon Taylor**, *New York Times* best-selling author of *Choices and Illusions*

*"Well, he has done it again! Dr. Norm Shealy continues to surprise me! He always has something new to present to the world. In this new book, **Living Bliss**, he takes healing to the heart of life, which is love. Read this, work with the suggestions, and be ready to travel the road to bliss."*
— **Gladys Taylor McGarey, M.D.**, past president of the American Holistic Medical Association and author of *Born to Heal*

"During the last ten years, I've been treating select patients with Norm Shealy's ring combinations along with acupuncture needles with gratifying results in most cases. Now that he has formulated and bottled specific aroma combinations for each ring, I have turned the treatments over to the patients themselves, starting with my wife. I can confirm from both personal and professional experience that stimulating these point combinations with the oils delivers the impact for which they are indicated. Thank you, Norm, for yet another remarkable and creative contribution to the evolution of modern medicine."

— **Joseph M. Helms, M.D.**, founding president,
American Academy of Medical Acupuncture;
president, Helms Medical Institute

"As one of the greatest innovative scholars of modern medicine, Dr. Norm Shealy shares with us his detailed and exciting journey to find relief for many of the world's most challenging diseases: depression, addiction, autism, PTSD, and multiple sclerosis.

"His innate willingness to follow his intuition and go where others fear to tread is credited to the fact that he truly cares about his patients and the advancement of medical science. This gift to the world could change your life forever."

— **Christine Page, M.D.**, author of *Frontiers of Health*

"In the 40 years that I have known Dr. C. Norman Shealy, I have never ceased to be awed by his tireless devotion to his mission of bringing about surcease of pain and suffering. Over those years, I have interviewed Norm for a number of magazines and for inclusion in my books. I have followed his research in pain clinics and in the examination of healers such as Henry Rucker and Olga Worrall. When I think of the long list of potions and instruments that Norm has created, there are times when he has seemed to me to be a kind of modern-day alchemist dedicated to the transformation of illness into wellness. Now, in this remarkable book, Dr. Shealy shares his passions, enthusiasms, and goals, and he challenges his readers to achieve their own betterment. With complete openness, he discloses the guidance of his angelic teacher and the inspiration that he has gained from *glimpses into his past lives. Of primary importance, we learn the value of being conscientious in every aspect of our life path. To emphasize the essential truth of this virtue, Dr. Shealy dedicates* **Living Bliss** *to his late beloved wife, Mary-Charlotte, 'the most conscientious person' he has ever known."*

— **Brad Steiger**, author of *Mysteries of Time and Space* and numerous other books on the paranormal and the unknown

"The year 2013 was quite possibly the most productive to date of Norm Shealy's most productive life. Early in the year he endowed a chair in conscientious psychology in a fully accredited university (Missouri State University) that assures serious attention for decades to come to a new branch of transpersonal psychology he and his wife, Chardy, explored. Later in the year he put the finishing touches on this, his most important book to date. To improve the quality of your life, consider the implications of conscientious psychology and try some of the treatments in this amazing book on bliss, entitled **Living Bliss!** *Thanks, Norm, for both the chair and the book."*

— **Bob Nunley, Ph.D.**, dean, Holos University
Graduate Seminary

Living
Bliss

ALSO BY C. NORMAN SHEALY MD, PhD

Alternative Medicine

The Complete Family Guide to Alternative Medicine

The Complete Illustrated Guide to Natural Home Remedies
(with Karen Sullivan)

The Directory of Complementary Therapies

Energy Medicine

The Healing Remedies Sourcebook

Holy Water, Sacred Oil

The Illustrated Encyclopedia of Healing Remedies

Life Beyond 100

Medical Intuition

The Methuselah Potential for Health and Longevity

Miracles Do Happen

Natural Progesterone Cream

90 Days to Self-Health

90 Days to Stress-Free Living

The Pain Game

Sacred Healing

The Self-Healing Workbook

Third Party Rape

To Parent or Not?

Living Bliss

Major Discoveries Along the Holistic Path

C. Norman Shealy MD, PhD

HAY HOUSE

Carlsbad, California • New York City • London • Sydney
Johannesburg • Vancouver • Hong Kong • New Delhi

First published and distributed in the United Kingdom by:
Hay House UK Ltd, Astley House, 33 Notting Hill Gate, London W11 3JQ
Tel: +44 (0)20 3675 2450; Fax: +44 (0)20 3675 2451
www.hayhouse.co.uk

Published and distributed in the United States of America by:
Hay House Inc., PO Box 5100, Carlsbad, CA 92018-5100
Tel: (1) 760 431 7695 or (800) 654 5126
Fax: (1) 760 431 6948 or (800) 650 5115
www.hayhouse.com

Published and distributed in Australia by:
Hay House Australia Ltd, 18/36 Ralph St, Alexandria NSW 2015
Tel: (61) 2 9669 4299; Fax: (61) 2 9669 4144
www.hayhouse.com.au

Published and distributed in the Republic of South Africa by:
Hay House SA (Pty) Ltd, PO Box 990, Witkoppen 2068
Tel/Fax: (27) 11 467 8904
www.hayhouse.co.za

Published and distributed in India by:
Hay House Publishers India, Muskaan Complex, Plot No.3, B-2,
Vasant Kunj, New Delhi 110 070
Tel: (91) 11 4176 1620; Fax: (91) 11 4176 1630
www.hayhouse.co.in

Distributed in Canada by:
Raincoast Books, 2440 Viking Way, Richmond, B.C. V6V 1N2
Tel: (1) 604 448 7100; Fax: (1) 604 270 7161; www.raincoast.com

Cover design: Angela Moody • *Interior design:* Bryn Starr Best
Interior photos/illustrations: Stephens Photography

The information given in this book should not be treated as a substitute for professional medical advice; always consult a medical practitioner. Any use of information in this book is at the reader's discretion and risk. Neither the author nor the publisher can be held responsible for any loss, claim or damage arising out of the use, or misuse, of the suggestions made, the failure to take medical advice or for any material on third party websites.

A catalogue record for this book is available from the British Library.

ISBN: 978-1-78180-305-9

Printed and bound in Great Britain by TJ International, Padstow, Cornwall.

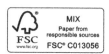

Dedicated to
Mary-Charlotte Bayles Shealy,
the most conscientious
person I have known.
Her inspiration has been
the light for my creativity.

CONTENTS

FOREWORD

by Caroline Myss

It's not a simple task to clear a new pathway in a familiar forest, but that's exactly what Norm Shealy has accomplished with this new book by introducing a word not often considered in the health arena: *conscientious.* As every reader will discover within the opening pages, this word comes with a substantial cache of power skills. It is not an ordinary word. Labeling a person as "conscientious" is a compliment that recognizes him or her as organized, reliable, dependable, and highly responsible. It took Norm's genius to focus on this particular power attribute in order that it might be recognized as having a core influence upon an individual's quality of life and health.

We have for decades written about, lectured on, and discussed at great length what it means to take personal responsibility for oneself in life. People are always saying, "I have to own that I did or said that," and such statements are accepted as admissions of responsibility. We have highlighted responsibility because over the course of the past six decades we have placed an increasing emphasis on the power the individual has to determine the quality of his or her life, health, and healing.

After reading this book, I felt that Norm had accomplished a milestone in terms of offering readers a much-needed guide in how to advance our understanding of responsibility; that is, there is a profound difference between the vague concept of wanting to live more responsibly and actually having a handbook that offers a person the essential directives on *how* to accomplish that goal. He has identified this life-changing choice as the decision to live a *conscientious life*. This has far-reaching benefits to an individual, as Norm points out in this wonderful book, not the least of which is that a conscientious person is more likely to live a happier as well as healthier lifestyle. As the reader will discover in the chapters of this book, Norm envisions health as inclusive of every element within our living environment.

Having taught in the field of consciousness and health studies for almost 30 years, I can honestly say that I have rarely heard mention of the word *conscientious* at all, much less used as a power skill. I have not, for example, ever done an intuitive reading and later told the person that he or she was depleted energetically as a result of living an "unconscientious" life. I have, however, suggested to many people throughout the years that they felt ungrounded. In general, the symptoms of someone who is ungrounded are these: unable to fulfill professional or personal commitments, difficulty with handling finances and often ending up in debt, the tendency to be renters and not landowners, the tendency to make endless promises but keep very few, and little capacity or desire to grasp the serious consequences generated by their lack of being grounded.

It is often especially challenging for ungrounded individuals to follow through with a creative idea, though not for lack of talent or genius. Rather, they find waiting for anything a near impossible task. Everything must happen now, all at once, or they move on. This is the same pattern of instant gratification that they bring to relationships, which explains why a long-term commitment with an ungrounded person usually ends in heartache.

We can agree that being ungrounded is obviously a challenge, an obstacle to a person's health and happiness. And to be clear, being ungrounded is not a choice. I think it is important to note that this particular type of "psychic suffering" is relatively new to the human experience. That is, more and more people today either feel completely ungrounded or go through periods in their life when they feel as if they have been uprooted from familiar earth. We are, in other words, experiencing new health challenges not only in the form of viruses such as HIV, but also in how we experience inner turmoil.

Looking back, I wish I'd had Norm's book as a guide to hand to these many individuals who knew they had a problem with being ungrounded but could not figure out how to navigate a positive route into a more stable emotional and psychic state. If any of them asked me now, "How do I break through this pattern of just quitting all the time?" I would hand them this book. I would introduce them to the idea of becoming a more conscientious person. Even as I write this, such a suggestion strikes me as a gentle and compassionate response, wise and nonthreatening. Norm has, in effect, written the perfect guidebook for people who feel as if they are disconnected from their physical or creative skills, or even their common sense. He has provided a type of anchoring system for individuals going through ungrounded cycles in life, which happens to all of us. We are living in a different world now, essentially a psychic one. Being "grounded" will soon become a standard setting on the medical dial.

I find that once again with this book, Norm has broken new ground. He never ceases to amaze me. I am sure that he will have that effect on you, too.

Caroline Myss,
Oak Park, IL
March 2013

∽∽∽ ∽∽∽

.

CHAPTER ONE

PRESENTING THE ROOTS OF CONSCIENTIOUS PSYCHOLOGY

If you felt loved and nurtured from the moment you entered this world, then you most likely grew up feeling fairly self-confident and secure within yourself. However, if you missed out on the nurturing you needed as a newborn baby or young child, I believe you can still heal and grow strong—through conscientiousness—and it's actually easier than you might think.

For more than 40 years as a neurosurgeon and holistic medical doctor, I have worked with 30,000 patients who came to me suffering with chronic pain and its insidious constant companion—depression. Through drive, determination, and an openness to try new things, I developed the most complete treatment plan I know of in the world. My patients—many of whom hobbled into the clinic doubled over in pain, wracked with anxiety, and often addicted to the drugs they were on—walked out with a new lease on life.

Within the Shealy pain clinic, we had an 85 percent success rate in treating patients who had been written off by the rest of the medical community! Six months later, we would follow up, and these people would still be functioning well—with little or no medications—able to do for themselves and for others. I still hear from past patients who have stayed in touch and who write to thank me for giving them their lives back.

The unique and comprehensive approach that helped them return to health and well-being has been continuously streamlined and documented through research papers, books, and newsletters I have written over the years. What once took months of inpatient care and therapy to accomplish is now available for individuals to read and learn—and it's geared toward those of you who agree that you don't want to live half a life anymore.

The people who have followed my radio call-in show for the past two decades every week in Missouri already know many of the techniques, therapies, and products that I have developed for optimal health and well-being. But now that wisdom and my own unique journey through the pain landscape are all in one place within this book, just in time to help you free yourself from illness, pain, depression, or despair.

It can be done—if you will but follow along and take action.

Developing a Conscientious Life

So if the steps themselves are easy enough to follow, you might wonder why so few people choose to lead a purposeful and conscientious life. Believe me, I've wondered that myself for over 40 years! And I've asked my patients, "What would it take for you to choose healthy habits?"

I have received a few good answers, but the majority of individuals just do not respond. They don't know what to say. And in my experience and through the extensive research I have done, the statistics also agree: About 97 percent of people do not even follow the four most basic health habits.

First, for too many people, they are carrying too much weight for their frame, and their body mass index (BMI) is too high. Your BMI should be between 18 and 24, but only about one-third of people achieve this. The second critical bad habit is smoking, which about 26 percent of Americans still do, even in this day and age. Third, only one-quarter of us eat at least five servings of fruit or vegetables daily. And fourth, only about 10 percent of us actually exercise a minimum of 30 minutes a day, five days a week.

So my suggested lifestyle adjustments incorporate these elements and a few other crucial steps that are geared to keep your body, mind, and spirit in top shape. You will see as we move along through this discussion that health and longevity are also served well by getting adequate sleep, keeping a positive attitude, developing a good social network, and taking about 20 minutes each day to develop your own spiritual foundation for life. Oh, and sex is good for you, too—how could I forget that? Just about everyone seems to enjoy that one!

These are all ways to live longer and healthier lives. I like to call them "bliss enhancers"—ways to raise the level of bliss you experience in this life. And as you read on and come to understand how all of this works, I will tell you about another route to bliss—a route that is even easier and faster, one that will jumpstart you on your path from illness and depression to a brighter existence in this world.

So How Do I Know What I Know?

Perhaps this advice seems rather simplistic and you've heard it before. Your parents, your grade-school gym teacher, your doctor, and just about every self-help book out there will point out many of these same techniques. There is a ton of data out there; we know that for sure. Do you need yet another book or expert to tell you to get off the couch and get with it?

I would say yes. If you are not enjoying a full and happy life, being good to yourself and others, and free of pain and depression, then something is wrong, and you are still missing a critical message. Or maybe some of your loved ones are suffering and unable to release themselves from the pain, fear, and anguish they feel each day. If you worry that you might die young or that your final years on this earth might be spent suffering with illness or senility, this is the time to read on and take this advice to heart.

I happen to know this topic inside out. From birth I was cut out for this exact path. One of the great gifts I received in this life is the parents I chose. They did not indoctrinate me with rigid beliefs that serve to strangle creativity. I was encouraged from a very young age to seek and understand the multidimensional reality of life.

And that I did! I soaked up learning from anywhere and everywhere—first from all my grade-school and high-school teachers, leaving with my diploma at 16 and heading to university. Then I learned from my professors and clinical training at some of the best medical facilities in the country when I was just barely 19 years old. Later I had to learn some rather brutal lessons during my neurosurgery residency, but that was short lived and I moved on as soon as I could.

Fortunately, along the way I had the most amazing mentors, too—consummate professionals who answered, and challenged, and supported me. Then, when I was working in different hospitals and within my own chronic-pain practice, I learned from my patients, listening to them and really trying to get at what was wrong and how we would and could fix it. I had to believe we could cure the kind of chronic pain that we were seeing. It was frustrating though; I had devoted my whole career to the study of pain, and yet people were still suffering.

Testing Medical Insight from Any and All Sources

As my world continued to open up, my own spiritual awakening began in earnest. I was fortunate to be on the leading edge of the holistic medical movement in America, which was also growing around the world in the 1970s. Suddenly there were no barriers to the world of health—it was not just surgery and drugs that I as a physician had to offer, but a whole range of new therapies and natural health products that were springing up everywhere. Many were based on the wisdom of the ages, but some practitioners were too crazy for words (for example, those who drank herbal tea, sang

"Kumbaya," and expected to cure themselves or others with feathers or some other such thing; I stayed well away from them!).

But I was drawn to the new ideas I was finding that seemed to have merit. I'd already tried and used the theories that the acupuncture field had presented, but I was later introduced to autogenic training (AT), behavior-modification theories, past-life therapy, and various kinds of supplements for the elements that our bodies seemed to need but were lacking.

I was in a unique situation to be able to test these new modalities and supplements in a clinical setting, in a safe and measured way, with patients who had tried everything else and were still unable to function due to excruciating pain and debilitating depression.

I also met some of the world's most incredible and accurate medical intuitives, and I realized I had that gift, too—when it first happened early in medical school I was chastised for it—but I later learned that many others also had this gift, and it was called *medical intuition.*

My first experience of it was during my sophomore year of medical school in physical-diagnosis class. We were asked to examine a patient and write up the diagnosis without asking the patient any questions. Intuitively, I made a correct diagnosis, but the doctor overseeing us accused me of cheating. He said that we should not have been able to make the diagnosis based solely on the physical exam. Then he said he would write up a highly critical report for my student file.

In my junior year, I wrote a 19-page history, physical exam, and diagnostic impression on a patient who came in over the weekend. I diagnosed the person with sarcoidosis of the pituitary gland. When I presented the case to the chief of endocrinology, he exclaimed, "You're a junior medical student. You can't make that diagnosis!" But I was correct, and he and I wrote a definitive paper on sarcoidosis of the hypothalamic-pituitary system.

Finding New Ways to Cure the Body, Mind, and Spirit

Later in my professional career, I often found that I was able to see beyond what the rest of the world sees—to know intuitively what was wrong with someone or suddenly understand how a new sort of therapy could work or what to try next. My scientific background in research, both in the lab and clinical settings, allowed me to construct tests of the various new ideas and keep adjusting them until we found what truly worked.

I also returned to school to take my Ph.D. in humanistic psychology, because more and more of my clinical-practice work seemed to be involved with curing matters of the mind and spirit, not just the physical body. The more I learned about how it all intertwined, the more I wanted to know. I just kept learning, as I still do today!

So that's how I have come to know what I know—but that is just the broadest of overviews. As you read along, and I explain further about the development of my own life path and about how conscientiousness has served me and those around me, these and other matters will become clearer.

I know that once you apply this knowledge and reach the ultimate goal of caring for yourself adequately, you will have ample energy, *and even a strong need,* to help others. Regardless of the circumstances of your birth or early years, you can overcome your past. Even those who suffered abuse or abandonment during their childhood or in their adult lives can be helped.

That is the purpose of this book. As you proceed through it with me, I will help you understand the concept of conscientiousness. In addition, I will describe practical ways in which you can improve yourself and significantly increase your own health and well-being—while also laying the foundation for your own psychology of conscientiousness. All you have to agree to right now is "I want to know more because I want a better life."

❦ ❦ ❦ ❦ ❦ ❦

CHAPTER TWO

The Makings of a Conscientious Life

Living and Breathing Conscientiousness

If you had ever met my wife, Mary-Charlotte, and spent any amount of time in her presence, you would have known what conscientiousness means. Chardy, as all her friends called her, embodied the essence of this personality trait, something I knew from the moment I met her. We had our first date on my 26th birthday, and I knew my search for the right mate was over!

Chardy was clearly the perfect match for me. She was conscientiousness personified, and she had so many wonderful qualities that I adored, such as her love for animals, beautiful singing voice, intelligence, and quiet elegance. Plus she was willing to put up with me and fully support all my activities and professional aspirations—what more could I want? We both wanted children, and we carefully planned for them. Our lives unfolded with love and without too much drama until 2010, when things suddenly shattered.

We had been married for more than 50 incredible years and saw no reason why we would not live to enjoy another 50! We both took excellent care of ourselves; we were conscientious about our health, embraced all aspects of a holistic lifestyle, ate an almost perfect diet, exercised, took supplements when needed, and basically followed all the steps that I knew were right for a long and healthy life. We were continuing to enjoy happy and healthy lives with our horses and other animals on our farm just outside of Springfield, Missouri.

What a shock when we found out that Chardy's genetic predisposition to myelodysplasia had caught up with her. Her father, her grandmother, and an uncle all experienced similar problems, but still we did not expect such a dire prognosis as she received in 2010—the doctors expected that she would live only another few months! She had developed acute myelogenous leukemia (AML), which evolved from myelodysplasia.

I knew from my career as a doctor and being active in medical research that even though we can control 75 percent of the factors impacting health and longevity through conscientious living, when faced with the reality of our genetics (which controls the other 25 percent), we can't always change the overall outcome.

This was the case with my beloved Chardy. Despite our best efforts and her own courageous fight, she could not beat it. They gave her only 3 months, but she fought it for 13. When she passed over, a part of me went with her.

Moving On Proved Harder Than Imagined

In 1994, I had a remarkable experience while on a holistic retreat; I felt my heart chakra fully open, and from that point on I understood more about love than I could ever comprehend before. I see now that this spiritual opening was a particularly important gift, because it helped me immensely as I tried to deal with my grief in losing Chardy—a reality that has been far more intense than I could have ever anticipated.

In the time since her death in 2011, I have cried more than in the first 77 years of my life. I discovered in a very personal way the true value of the many therapies and products that I developed over the years to help my patients overcome pain, depression, and loss. When I turned to these same techniques, they helped me immensely. For example, I have used my Liss Cranial Stimulator (LCS) more since her death than during the entire previous 25 years, and I use the Air Bliss essential oils blend daily, which I know is one of the main reasons that I have been able to go on without her.

I will fully explain these products and therapies in the coming chapters, because that's what this book is all about. But first, in order to understand all of that, I feel it is crucial for you to first know why conscientiousness is so important and how boosting certain hormones and biochemical processes in the body can help bring out greater self-love and self-care. This has been a long journey of discovery for me, and one that I am very happy to share, because I know it will change your life.

Why Should You Strive to Be Conscientious?

The study of conscientiousness by psychologists goes back decades. Conscientiousness is one of the big five personality traits, according to psychologists. Specifically, the five sets of traits that psychologists like to measure are: extroverted vs. introverted, agreeable vs. antagonistic, conscientious vs. unfocused, neurotic vs. emotionally stable, and open to experience vs. not open to experience. For our purposes, we are going to concentrate primarily on conscientiousness.

What is it that conscientious people care about, and why should you care? Well, these individuals are pretty easy to recognize. They are prepared, neat, and orderly. They like things scheduled, and they approach tasks in a focused, organized, and disciplined manner. Conscientious individuals are careful, thorough, reliable, persistent, and prudent; it may sound a bit boring to some of you, but all these traits are good to have if you want to live a long and healthy life. Conscientious people are particularly resilient when life gives them big challenges that must be faced.

But the most critical aspect of conscientiousness is responsibility; they do not blame others for their own problems. It is responsibility for self that is the cornerstone, and it leads a person to become stronger in all other aspects of conscientiousness.

Not surprisingly, conscientious individuals achieve high levels of success by starting with purposeful planning and persistence and the knowledge for how to learn from their mistakes. They know that they need to process their life experiences in order to extract the big lessons, and they also know how to flush out the residue.

I believe that in the same way we process food when we eat, we also need to chew up our experiences. We need to sort them out to understand what has happened to us and why. This allows us to digest the real substance and extract what we need to learn. Through reflection of our experiences, we assimilate wisdom and insight, and in turn we can revise our beliefs, priorities, and methods continuously. As we do that, we can flush out what is left over, the residue, or *irritation.*

This concept of *irritation* came to me from Torkom Saraydarian, an American teacher, author, and spiritualist who said in his wonderful booklet that irritation destroys the etheric nervous system, while also listing almost 30 "causes" of irritation. In other words, you cannot afford the luxury of anger, guilt, anxiety, or depression!

To be conscientious in this sense means to discern thoroughly and skillfully your life experiences and apply what you have learned. This makes real growth in life possible. It also gives us the capacity to recognize our responsibilities and manage them in a practical and effective manner.

However, many people are just the opposite of conscientious. They are the ones who don't know how to take personal responsibility and are quick to blame anyone and everyone else, even society or the universe, for the misery that they face. You quite likely know a person like this—probably quite a few. It's never their fault that they don't have a good job, their spouse left them, or they have this nagging back pain that sidelines them from life.

During my career, I have met thousands of these kinds of souls, and I would say that virtually all of them were depressed. I have devoted my entire career, some 40 years, to the researching and perfecting of techniques that would allow these individuals to overcome depression, recover from chronic pain, and live longer and healthier lives than even modern medicine would expect. One of the main keys to this puzzle was the study of dehydroepiandrosterone (DHEA), and that is where we're going next.

Discovering the Amazing Role of DHEA

One of the most important "aha" moments in my whole career was when I realized that there was a way to raise the levels of DHEA naturally in our bodies—not just one way, but four ways. This was something that no one had known was possible before this point.

This was a very important discovery, because DHEA is produced naturally in the human body and is the most abundant circulating steroid we have. Optimal health requires optimal levels of DHEA, but these levels in the body begin to decrease naturally after age 30.

DHEA is produced in the adrenal glands, the testicles, and the brain. In the human body, it functions predominantly as a metabolic intermediate in the creation of the male and female sex steroids.

It has been used by doctors as a treatment for some conditions, such as adrenal insufficiency and depression, but no studies of long-term supplement effects have been conducted. It is suspected that taking DHEA can cause higher-than-normal levels of androgens and estrogens in the body, and theoretically this may increase the incidence of some cancers. Therefore, taking DHEA as an oral treatment is not without risk, and so I asked myself, "Is there some other natural way we could encourage our bodies to increase DHEA levels?"

My quest for this discovery became the number one priority of my research efforts in the early 1990s, since I was working with thousands of depressed, pain-filled patients and wondering what would help them the most. While seeking answers, I developed the concept of neurochemical profiling, which is a critical diagnostic system for depression.

With neurochemical profiling, I set out to measure the levels of various neurochemicals in the body through inspecting spinal fluid or blood. That's when I found out that 100 percent of my patients who had chronic pain and depression were deficient in DHEA! One hundred percent!

Overcoming Deficiencies Within Our Bodies

While researching DHEA, I found many other deficiencies as well. In fact, when I looked at the 10 essential amino acids in the human body, patients seemed to be deficient in one or most of these or their optimal ratios were not in balance, which I suspected we needed to resolve.

For example, at this time I also discovered that 84 percent of depressed patients were deficient in taurine and 100 percent of them were deficient in intracellular magnesium, but those cases were a little easier to understand and alleviate. Both taurine and magnesium are critical in maintaining the electrical charge on cells, and taurine is now considered "conditionally essential" for the human body. Interestingly, it is present *only* in animal protein. There is no taurine in any vegetable. While my patients did usually eat meat, they seemed to neither digest nor absorb the animal protein or they somehow had an increased need for taurine. Fortunately, it is available as a supplement.

As for treating the magnesium deficiency, I found that rather than take an oral magnesium supplement, patients actually got a far better and quicker benefit by using magnesium lotion and rubbing it directly on their skin twice daily. When I was testing these theories, I also developed many other techniques and therapies to help treat these same depressed patients, which I will talk more about in the coming chapters.

But I'd like to return now to the DHEA discussion, because it is still the most critical hormone in the body for determining health. Through my research, I discovered four natural methods of rejuvenating the body's ability to make DHEA. I found that each of the four techniques would have its own incremental effect on raising levels, but no single innovation seemed to be able to do it all on its own.

The four natural methods to raise levels of DHEA in the body that I discovered were these: using natural progesterone cream, taking a specific vitamin-mineral complex that I developed called Youth Formula, applying magnesium lotion to the skin, and activating a series of points on the body that correspond to the Ring of Fire (this is one of five Sacred Rings that is explained in more detail in Chapter Seven). Research also indicates that levels of DHEA in our bodies are naturally enhanced when we are experiencing joy, having sex, and spending time out in the sunshine, but of course it's rather hard to measure the exact benefits in those cases.

By the way, my first intuitive hit for DHEA restoration was to use natural progesterone cream. This idea came to me as an inspiration, and it worked. Many of my new ideas—I guess virtually all of them—seem to be downloaded into my brain from divine guidance, and then I have been fortunate to be able to use my medical training and research capacity to study these ideas further in order to prove or perfect them.

So What Has Made You What You Are?

I'd like to return now to the discussion about personality, because it helps explain why some people are conscientious in their approach to life and others are not. It has been commonly accepted that personality and mood are conditioned by many different factors, such as your genetic makeup and your environment, and many people believe your birth order, your astrological sign, or even karma play a role.

But there is a growing body of knowledge that says that our emotional environment during gestation (when we were in our mother's womb) and the moment of birth may well be more critical than all the other factors combined!

Research is showing us that these factors, occurring from the very moment of conception to age seven, help to determine the personality and mood of a person. And once that early foundation is created, it is difficult to change—not impossible, but it takes effort.

Here's how it works: The human baby about to be born has an oxytocin system that is ready and waiting to be activated, and that burst of oxytocin is conditioned to happen naturally at birth. (Oxytocin is the nurturing, bonding hormone that is so vital to our lives.) This burst of oxytocin from the mother sets the child up to bond naturally with the mother and allows the child to form a healthy attachment that will serve the child well as he or she begins a new life on Earth.

However, when the mother undergoes any kind of trauma while pregnant or while giving birth, it can and does impact the child. For example, when a mother undergoes a Cesarean section to deliver the child by surgery, the natural surge or burst of oxytocin is not delivered to the baby the way it would happen through the natural process of birth. Likewise, if women are given artificial oxytocin (in the form of Pitocin) to induce delivery, that can also prevent the child from getting that natural burst of oxytocin.

We also know that if any kind of major trauma happens in the first seven years of life, a child's oxytocin mechanism can shut down. Any kind of abuse, whether it is physical, sexual, emotional, or verbal, can cause trauma to the child, as can parental divorce. While divorce is not obviously abusive, it more often than not interrupts the nurturing process. So while the children of divorce are not in any physical danger, they might not feel as safe and secure as they once did, if they lived with two loving parents.

But whenever a person of any age who has healthy levels of oxytocin enjoys a happy, nurturing episode, it causes the emotional center of that person to say, "Hey, that feels good," because a burst of oxytocin is released. The person enjoys a warm feeling of comfort and happiness. Oxytocin also brings out increased optimism, and the hormone acts as a powerful modulator of social behaviors. It also modulates the release of serotonin, which is one of the body's most critical mood chemicals.

Even young children who are secure and happy on a daily basis exhibit conscientious traits, and if those traits or actions are encouraged, modeled, or rewarded, the young ones become even more conscientious as they mature. However, if they have not had the reinforcement of the bonding experience at birth, and in the first seven years have not felt a sufficient level of self-esteem, they will feel this lack throughout their lives.

Here is another example: If one or both parents are not fully approving of their son or daughter, as might be the case if mom and dad chastise the child because his or her test scores at school were not good enough, the child's self-esteem might resultantly be damaged. Now, it should be pointed out that this does not cause as much damage as physical abuse, but parents being overly critical can, and very often do, create doubt in their children as to their own self-worth. By the time kids reach their teenage years, most personality problems they may exhibit can be directly linked to a deficiency in oxytocin.

The bottom line is that the quantity and quality of the nurturing you got during the first seven years of life determined to a great degree the level of social competence you have as an adult and your ability to cope with stress and aggressiveness.

Too Little Oxytocin Can Cause Big Problems

In addition to being a primary factor in poor self-esteem, there is a huge body of evidence indicating that oxytocin deficiency influences a wide spectrum of disorders, including autism, attention deficit/hyperactivity disorder (ADHD), depression, obsessive-compulsive disorder (OCD), borderline personality, addiction, and schizophrenia.

In fact, almost all psychotherapy from the past 200 years has been related to these problems. I feel shock and dismay when I think that therapists have been attempting to change personality within their patients without resetting the thermostat that actually controls it—which is oxytocin!

That's why I am suggesting that a different approach is needed. While I fully accept that nutritional factors, social circumstances, and environmental conditions are all part of the picture of how we turn into functioning adults in our society, I also believe that boosting oxytocin actually has the potential to make a far greater impact and improvement on our lives than just about anything else.

Although the full effects of boosting oxytocin have not yet been studied in the long term, the results seen in the past ten years, for example, are far more striking than any other single intervention. So far, the main way of increasing oxytocin in the body is to take it via a nasal spray.

I have found more than 20 references to the power and effectiveness of oxytocin, which I have included in the bibliography. Many of those studies have shown, for instance, that acute intranasal oxytocin improves positive self-perceptions of personality and reduces social anxiety and fear.

Raising oxytocin levels through a nasal spray, however, is somewhat cumbersome, and I believe this spray would be very hard on sensitive nasal membranes if used for extended periods of time. But since we know now that oxytocin does work, my approach was to find natural ways to increase oxytocin levels. And so I have.

Understanding Oxytocin and Its Power

While I have worked with DHEA for more than 20 years, I became aware of the recent oxytocin studies only a few months after Chardy's death in 2011. I happened to find a few articles on oxytocin, and I knew instantly that this had to be another divine inspiration knocking on my door. I felt pretty strongly that the therapies I had been developing that were increasing neurotensin, critical for reducing stress, in the body must also raise levels of oxytocin. But how was I to be sure?

This was such a new topic that I had difficulty finding very much credible research. I spent hours on the Internet and finally found a research paper reporting that oxytocin is released when neurotensin increases. I knew it! I was so excited that I actually had difficulty sleeping that night. At this point, I already knew that one of the therapies I'd developed allowed the body to increase its production of neurotensin; now I knew that that particular approach would also allow the body to raise its level of oxytocin in the same natural way.

This is particularly good news if you are one of the individuals who did not feel as loved, wanted, or nurtured from birth onward as you should have been. If you experienced trauma in your early years, or even on your way through life as an adult, it is not too late. Anyone suffering from post-traumatic stress disorder (PTSD) can be helped. You can learn to nurture yourself by becoming more conscientious and also take steps to restore your oxytocin capacity. It is very important that you feel lovable and loved; everyone requires this.

Not only that, but oxytocin is also a major stress reducer. It's important to humans because healthy functioning of your oxytocin system positively influences social behavior, social affiliations, and memory, while also helping to control anxiety, mood, and the tendency to overeat. Oxytocin also moderates fear by inhibiting the adrenocorticotropic hormone (ACTH) and the release of cortisone. In other words, oxytocin is a natural antidepressant.

The Next Logical Step—Doing Good for Self and Others

There is another extremely important aspect of conscientiousness that I don't want to leave out. It is related to the age-old debate about our purpose on Earth, the meaning of life. I was almost 40 years old when I figured this out. Simply put, I believe that our only *purpose* in life is to learn how to fulfill our greatest basic human instinct, and that is *to help other people.*

My premise is that if we felt adequately nurtured as children, then we will naturally feel this need as adults, clearly hearing and heeding the call to do good for ourselves and others. This awareness grows within us as we mature. However, if we weren't adequately nurtured as children, we need to do that for ourselves now: nurture ourselves so we can then help ourselves and others.

This book gives you the understanding and the tools to boost your good feelings about yourself, regardless of where you are in life. Once you know how good you are and how much better life can be, then you will be ready to fulfill your primary purpose of helping other people.

Why Not Choose to Experience a Blissful Life?

Suppose I could give you an elixir of health and well-being. Not one you would drink, but one that you could apply to specific points on your body in just 30 seconds.

Suppose you could use specific elixirs to increase DHEA, which we know is the most important hormone in your body. What if you could activate calcitonin development in your body, which is essential for bone strength and pain control? Or perhaps you would like to reduce the scavenging effects of free radicals that essentially "rust" your body?

Of course, like so many people, you may just need a good surge of oxytocin, which helps you feel secure, happy, and at peace with yourself and the world.

Those elixirs are available now, and I describe them in detail in Chapter Seven. They have the capacity to help you rebuild your body's own natural functioning, but they are not a magic bullet. If you truly wish to change your life and achieve optimal health, happiness, and longevity, I challenge you now to embrace your inner conscientious self and keep reading along.

In the next few chapters, I will describe how I came to discover the wisdom I am sharing with you now, and explain how you can understand better and embrace your own spiritual power. Then I will present the practical lifestyle adjustments that you can make to pave your way to optimal health and longevity.

But first, let's look at a compelling research study that proves that conscientiousness is the first important skill you need to master. Without it, as you will soon see, life can take some pretty miserable turns.

ა ა ა   ა ა ა

CHAPTER THREE

RESEARCH LINKING CONSCIENTIOUSNESS AND LONGEVITY

One of the most powerful studies explaining the impact of conscientiousness on human development came about through an extensive research project that began in 1921. The study lasted 80 years, and it culminated in a fascinating and comprehensive book titled *The Longevity Project* by Howard S. Friedman, Ph.D., and Leslie R. Martin, Ph.D.

In this chapter, I present some of the main highlights from Friedman and Martin's book, because their findings clearly make a compelling case for conscientiousness. In order to be truly healthy and have a long, happy life, you have to have conscientiousness. *The Longevity Project* study concluded that conscientiousness is the single greatest factor for *health* and *longevity*. Incidentally, genes influence your health by only 25 percent.

As you will see here, many factors determine spontaneous conscientiousness. For example, having two married parents is the basic foundation; women are often more likely to have the conscientious personality trait than men; and, even though longevity is far less important than health, both longevity and health are affected by the same experiences.

You see, even if you live a conscientious life, like my beloved wife, that still isn't enough to avoid suffering from some diseases that shorten it. Two days after I finished reading Friedman and Martin's book, my wife of 52 years died. An agonizing 13-month battle ended. I decided then to devote my life to studying, teaching, and motivating others about conscientiousness.

I had already spent my whole career helping people overcome pain and depression. I saw time and time again that the real problem for at least 75 percent of people I treated was that they lacked healthy habits, and this was primarily due to poor self-esteem.

It was tremendously exciting for me to find another missing link in this puzzle in 2011 when I dug into *The Longevity Project* findings. It introduced me to the next logical step in my own research, and since then my efforts have been focused on exploring the field of conscientiousness and, specifically, conscientious psychology. So let me speak now about Friedman and Martin's findings, and you can see for yourself the powerful impact conscientiousness can have in your own life.

Studying the Impact of Conscientiousness on Human Development

The Longevity Project was an extensive and ambitious research project established in 1921 by Dr. Lewis Terman, who was an American psychologist and a noted pioneer in educational psychology in the early 20th century. Dr. Terman asked teachers to pick their "brightest" students, and just over 1,500 boys and girls, who were born around 1910, were selected for this 80-year-long study. Several groups of research scientists have since continued the work after Dr. Terman died in 1956.

The project concluded with the publication of the book I've just mentioned above: *The Longevity Project: Surprising Discoveries for Health and Long Life from the Landmark Eight-Decade Study.* I discovered this book through reading a review one day in the *New York Times* and was fascinated to read more.

Friedman and Martin's findings—the culmination of following the lives of these children, and eventually adults, for some 80 years—shed light on what truly contributes to a long and healthy life. Here are only two of the authors' conclusions: "Eating slowly doesn't much matter," and "Lying about your age and your health does indeed represent a challenge to health researchers."

The authors also proved that—surprise, surprise—people who live to ripe, old ages do so because they outlive most serious illnesses. Throughout their lives, the subjects who did live to the oldest ages tended to be happier than those who ended up dying younger. And, incidentally, the ones who lived longest also tended to be healthier.

Since, presumably, all people want to live happy and healthy lives well into their senior years and be physically sound and mentally alert right up to the end, do you know what else made the difference? Persistence and prudence.

These just happen to be two of the greatest qualities of conscientiousness and, therefore, the study proved that conscientiousness, when measured in childhood, is the best predictor of longevity. It is also the best personality predictor for long life when measured in adulthood. Related major qualities of conscientious people, such as thrift, being detail oriented, and living responsibly, were all seen to contribute to individuals leading longer and healthier lives.

As it turned out, by the year 2000, 70 percent of the women and 51 percent of the men who were determined to be conscientious in this study had died. The deceased were all born about 90 years earlier; however, it is important to note that the *less* conscientious of them *died much earlier.*

The reason for this is that conscientious people do more to protect their health. They engage in fewer risky activities. They're less likely to smoke, less likely to drink excessively, less likely to do drugs, and less likely to drive too fast. Conscientious people tend to take more safety precautions and are more likely to wear seat belts.

Friedman and Martin concluded that people are *biologically predisposed* to be both healthier and more conscientious. Furthermore, the researchers stated that serotonin is necessary "to regulate many health-relevant processes throughout the body, including how much you eat and how well you sleep." I knew from my research that individuals with low serotonin levels are more impulsive, and low serotonin is a major foundation of depression.

I found this very interesting, because low levels of oxytocin are another cause of low self-esteem. There is indeed a strong relationship between oxytocin and serotonin.

The Many Benefits of Living a Conscientious Life

Interestingly, conscientious people tend to seek healthier situations and relationships. They have happier marriages, better friendships, and healthier work situations. Friedman and Martin emphasized that these individuals make adjustments to their lives as others do, but they take smaller, more incremental steps—they avoid rapid and sudden changes.

On the other hand, the authors concluded that those who are less conscientious are more likely to be clinically depressed, feel anxious, smoke cigarettes, and have high blood pressure and sciatica—and also have tuberculosis, diabetes, joint problems, and strokes. While it was believed that these people can still lead exciting and very rewarding lives, nonetheless they may not feel as good as they could. As an active physician for 40-plus years, most of my clinical practice involved patients who needed help managing these exact problems.

Apparently, being an extrovert and sociable by itself does not necessarily increase longevity. This was something I knew from my own experience, but it was interesting to see it confirmed. Friedman and Martin approached it through looking at the personalities of scientists and engineers, who tend to be polar opposites of businessmen and lawyers in their abilities, occupational interests, and social behaviors. But generally speaking, scientists outlived nonscientists. The findings in *The Longevity Project* concluded that only two-thirds of nonscientists reached age 70, but almost three-quarters of scientists did so, too.

Scientists in general tend to be less sociable than lawyers, businesspeople, and salespeople. Overall, the two groups are about equal in conscientiousness, but scientists tended to have long-lasting marriages and more stable jobs where they worked responsibly.

In contrast, nonscientists tended to have more tumultuous, less stable, and more health-damaging careers and behaviors. So sociability did not make someone healthier and allow them to live longer—or cause them to be conscientious in and of itself; it had to do with these other factors.

However, the authors did say that individuals who *as children* were more sociable and extroverted tended to drink and smoke more. In my experience with more than 30,000 depressed people (the majority of whom were introverts), I found that those who became invalids were the ones who were much more likely to be introverts and that they were far more likely to smoke than the extroverts.

Nonetheless, the authors state that length of life is the single best measure of health, and that cheerful and optimistic children are less likely to live to an old age than their more staid and sober counterparts. That's because overly cheerful children engaged in riskier hobbies and paid less conscious attention to their health.

The Effects of Conscientiousness Developed During Adulthood

Friedman and Martin emphasized repeatedly that adopting healthy habits, such as watching less TV, improving social relations, increasing activity, and helping others, was not as important as having these qualities innately. But it is entirely possible to develop increasing conscientiousness and even extroversion! I am a perfect example of someone who was strongly introverted until age 19 when I entered medical school. I intuited that I needed to become an extrovert, played the role for a few years, and have been extroverted for the past 60 years while remaining conscientious.

Conscientious people are also far less likely to be "catastrophizers" (otherwise known as people who make a mountain out of a molehill). Research has shown that those individuals—especially men—tend to die sooner. Catastrophizers are more likely to die from accidents or violence. During interviews with older men (those in the longevity study who lived until over the age of 70), not one of them ever spoke the word *death* in reference to his own inevitable demise.

Another interesting study illustrates this same point quite well. Individuals were given propranolol (a drug used to treat hypertension, anxiety, and panic) or a placebo, and the conscientious people were much more likely to survive whether they took the placebo or the drug. *In other words, the conscientiousness of taking it was more important than ingesting the drug itself!* I fully understand this happening, because I have seen this result more than once myself, where the conscientiousness of taking the medicine had a greater impact than whether the subject got the placebo or the drug.

In *The Longevity Project,* Friedman and Martin spoke often about the fact that the patterns of behavior in early childhood are far more important than any other single indicator of health. Although breast-feeding may have other benefits, they determined that it *did not* appear to affect personality. They did find, however, that a greater number of study participants who began school at a very early age encountered more difficulty throughout life and led shorter lives. Children who started first grade at age five were at a much higher risk of dying early than those who started at age six. Incidentally, I am happy to report personally being an exception to this finding and am still with you at age 80 to tell this story!

The Impact of Parental Divorce

You might expect individuals who have more education to live longer and healthier lives; however, the level of education by itself did not seem to be a good predictor of health or longevity. While society places huge value on getting the proper education, there was another life experience that was far more of a factor in the equation than what these children learned in school.

It turns out that one of the most critical life experiences these young people had to deal with was parental divorce. More than one-third of the Terman group faced either death of a mother or father or divorce of their parents. Death itself did not seem to impact the life span of that son or daughter, but "[t]he long-term health effects of parental divorce were often devastating—it was indeed a risky circumstance that changed the pathways of many of the young Terman participants."

I have found this to be true in so many cases within my clinical work that I was very much interested in these actual findings. In general, the final report concluded that "[c]hildren from divorced families died almost five years earlier on average than children from intact families." Parental divorce during childhood was "the single strongest social predictor of early death, many years into the future."

On the other hand, early childhood personality and the effects of parental divorce did not seem related. This is because there were many other independent factors that contributed to health, such as, for example, men were more likely than women to die early of accidents or of violence if their parents had divorced. In other words, they became more reckless.

Among other things, *The Longevity Project* showed that both boys and girls in divorced families had less long-term education. These children were more likely to engage in drinking and smoking—especially smoking—and women from broken homes were more than twice as likely to be heavy smokers. Sons and daughters from these households also had an increased risk of cancer, and they were much more likely to get divorced themselves.

The study also stressed what has been commonly accepted for a long time: Married men live longer. Divorced men have a much higher mortality risk, and less than one-third of divorced men reached age 70. However, the study also showed that married women did not necessarily live longer. Women who divorced their husbands and stayed single lived almost as long as steadily married women. This agrees with what I have seen in my clinical practice as well—that divorce is much *less harmful* to women's health than it is to men's.

From *The Longevity Project,* the women who grew up with parents who remained married were also less likely to become divorced. In terms of conscientiousness, the authors found that "folks who later became consistently married individuals had been more conscientious as children." In other words, prudence and responsibility as a child was more likely to lead to a successful marriage and longer life.

The Role of Exercise in Health and Longevity

With regard to exercise, *The Longevity Project* also concluded that "being active in middle age was most important to health and longevity." In other words, being inactive during childhood did not hinder health and longevity if the individual became more active as he or she aged. This I definitely agree with. Time and time again, I have seen adults of all ages overcome pain and depression more quickly and more consistently when they began to exercise in a conscientious way, regardless of early patterns.

On the flip side, *The Longevity Project* also showed that those who were active as children were more likely to remain active. However, if they became inactive as adults, then the protection of physical activity vanished. Friedman and Martin really emphasized that moderate exercise is significantly more important than running marathons or other vigorous, prolonged exercising.

Tracing the Impact on Career Progress and Success

Of the men in the Terman study, about 20 percent were considered highly successful and 20 percent unsuccessful. Sixty percent were in between successful and unsuccessful. What is important is that those who had the *greatest success* in their careers were *less likely* to die young. Put another way, the most successful men lived five years longer than the least successful.

The researchers stated it this way: "[A]mbition, coupled with perseverance, impulse control, and high motivation, was not only good for achievement but was part of the package of a resilient work life." Both work and family were the most important aspects for health and longevity for men. Males who worked more stressful jobs died younger, as you might expect.

But being happy in those stressful jobs doesn't necessarily matter for longevity. They say that a man's productive orientation means more to him than his social relationships or worrying about being personally happy. As with everything else, prudence, dependability, and perseverance seem to be real keys—conscientiousness wins again!

The Power of Actively Working Through Pain

There is a huge difference between chronic-pain patients who become invalids and those who continue to live their lives actively despite pain or even physical disability. Actor Christopher Reeve and well-known author and theoretical physicist Stephen Hawking are two examples of extraordinarily productive individuals despite both having some of the worst possible disabilities. Reeve became a quadriplegic after being thrown from a horse, and Hawking developed a motor neuron disease related to amyotrophic lateral sclerosis (ALS). I have found that individuals such as Reeve and Hawking, who really enjoy their work, rarely become invalids even when they have ongoing pain.

In comparison, a study from the 1970s showed that those who had preexisting personality problems, as suggested by the Minnesota Multiphasic Personality Inventory (MMPI), were far more likely to have chronic pain and disability after back surgery. And another study proved that smokers were nine times less likely to improve after back surgery than nonsmokers!

In fact, 75 percent of my chronic-pain patients had elevated scores on hysteria, depression, and hypochondriasis, and another 15 percent had elevated scores on even more serious personality traits, such as schizoid behavior, paranoia, and so on. After four or five years of routinely doing MMPI evaluations on all of my chronic-pain patients, I stopped, because it is so difficult to discuss such undesirable traits!

Instead, I started using the California Psychological Inventory (CPI), which measures 18 variables such as dominance, capacity for status, sociability, self-acceptance, independence, empathy, responsibility, socialization, and self-control. The traits measured by the CPI tool are remarkably important in evaluating conscientiousness, and I found it much easier to discuss excess or deficient behavior in any of them with my patients.

I also found out that chronic-pain patients who had become invalids had an average of 49 symptoms on my Total Symptom index, but to give you some perspective, anyone with 30 or more symptoms is highly stressed or terminally ill! (My patients have not generally been terminally ill.) Furthermore, on a Total Life Stress (TLS) test, my patients tended to average a score of 75 or above, and higher than 25 on the TLS is enough to increase the number of overall symptoms. In fact, my typical patient had an average of five significant diagnoses in addition to chronic pain. Clearly, people who have great stress also have a wide range of symptoms!

Spirituality, Social Networks, and Doing Good for Others

From these findings in my own practice, I determined that one of the best ways to alleviate pain was to get rid of stress. I also knew that, within the clinic, a good way to bring stress down was to get people more socially engaged—basically, encourage them to make friends and do things for others.

Therefore, I was very interested to read that *The Longevity Project* researchers also included a study of social engagement and the place of religion as factors that had an effect on health and longevity. They concluded that religiosity did not matter much for men, but it did for women. They also found that it wasn't *religion* itself, but rather other personality aspects that were more significant to women. The real importance of religion seemed to be in the activity of social networking—attending ceremonies, participating in community-welfare activities, and being involved in other various church functions.

In contrast, researchers found that for the men, their family and career were far more essential than religion. It was actually family and career social engagement that were more vital to them. In other words, the most crucial effects on health and longevity for both men and women appeared to be the frequency with which they visited and communicated with relatives, friends, and neighbors, and that they participated in community service and found satisfaction with friendships and social contacts.

Other important factors for both sexes included the number of intimate and companionate bonds they enjoyed with others, the quality of the relationships they had with family and close relatives, and how often they attended meetings with social or community groups.

This last point—participation in social or community groups—turned out to be perhaps the most fundamental of all. The authors continued their report by saying that although other studies have shown that those who feel loved and cared for will claim a better sense of well-being, they did not find that this helped much for living a longer life. But having a large social network mattered tremendously—even more so than playing with pets. Over and over, the participants emphasized that helping, advising, and caring for others were among the most powerful factors for men and women in leading longer and healthier lives.

I totally agree—and have seen this proven many times in my practice. People with chronic pain reported to me that just about every time they were asked what their desire to get better was, they said that they wanted to be able to help others. I believe that doing good for our fellow human beings is one of our most natural inclinations, and when an individual is wracked with pain or suffering from depression, he or she misses out on fulfilling this vital need. I find it telling, and very true, that according to Friedman and Martin, "[S]ocial relations should be the first place to look for improving health and longevity."

The Nonimpact of Modern Medical Advances on Longevity

Many people believe that physicians and their research are extending the human life span. However, *The Longevity Project* proved a point that I personally have always believed, namely that modern medical cures have actually played a relatively minor role in increasing the overall length of our lives. I know this is something that most people do not understand fully, but it's true. In fact, the average life expectancy of a 60-year-old white male in the United States has increased only 4 or 5 years during the past 50.

In the words of the *Longevity* authors, "It is a great misconception (with serious implications) in our society that modern medicine has led to huge increases in the longevity of American adults." Many other researchers concur with this finding, including Dr. Thomas McKeown in his book *The Role of Medicine,* which emphasized the fact that 92 percent of the increased longevity in the 20th century had nothing at all to do with medical advances. Furthermore, hundreds of articles, some even published in the *Journal of the American Medical Association,* listed the medical system itself as the third leading *cause* of death. Meanwhile, several others have said medical intervention is, by far, the *number one* cause of death!

Of course, as one might expect, depression, hostility, and aggressiveness all carry risks of a wide variety of illnesses, as well as shortened life expectancy. Friedman and Martin concluded that individual health depends on social health, and they also stated that "[r]esilience was not a trait they were born with, nor an inner insight, but a process of perseverance and hard work."

They also suggested that long life is associated with "an active pursuit of goals, a deep satisfaction of life, and a strong sense of accomplishment." They believe that you cannot predict how healthy you'll be or how long you'll live based on your parents' lives. It appears that the most important thing we can do to help people is to aid them in developing healthy social patterns and "inter-activity."

These findings certainly back up in a compelling way what I have always known: Conscientious people live longer and healthier lives because they take responsibility for themselves and for their actions each day. Simply put, they make sound choices. This was the premise for my own Ph.D. thesis in 1976 and the impetus for my best-selling book that came out of that research titled *90 Days to Self-Health*. Now my passion is to help everyone enjoy health and longevity through the power of conscientious living!

ᵕᵕᵕ ᵕᵕᵕ

CHAPTER FOUR

CLINICAL INNOVATIONS IN TACKLING CHRONIC PAIN AND DEPRESSION

I was only one year into my career as a neurosurgeon when I came to a life-changing realization. The most common symptom in the world was pain, and yet nobody seemed to be specializing in it. So at age 30, I decided that this is what the focus of my life would be: what causes it, what we can do about it, and how it affects us as human beings.

Pain turned out to be more than just a focus—it became my life's work, and I still wake up every day wondering what it is that we still need to know. Intrinsically linked to my study of pain is depression, which is a debilitating condition that my patients suffered from alongside the chronic pain.

As a young professional in this field, I was just starting to dig into the topic of pain management, when I quickly realized that most of the long-term fixes for chronic pain did not actually come from the established medical community, but rather from the domain of folk medicine. So I began a series of research studies that included any ideas I came across that were claiming to be able to treat chronic discomfort in the long term without the use of narcotics.

It led me into a fascinating new world that included cures put forward by acupuncturists, mystics, faith healers, color therapists, hypnotherapists, doctors of homeopathy, spiritual healers, and other nontraditional therapists. As I tested many various modalities and therapies, I came to the conclusion that while none of these methods was the single cure for chronic pain (the magic bullet, so to speak), almost all of them had some ability to eliminate it successfully in a majority of patients.

It was at this juncture I figured out that it must actually be the interaction of the four main fields of stress that causes illness in the body—those four being the chemical, mechanical, electromagnetic, and emotional fields. I soon knew with certainty that not only did the interactions of these fields cause some illnesses, but they caused all illnesses in the human body. *All!* Clearly I would have lots of work to do.

But overall I would say that my success within the pain clinic came about because I was able to blend the many holistic health concepts that worked with the knowledge I had from my traditional, mainstream medical training. It was this combination of science and metaphysics that allowed me to break so much new ground in the emerging field of pain management, and in turn the treatment of depression.

Depression is not well understood and can be defined in many ways. At the psychological level, it is much more than a feeling of sadness or discouragement. It also manifests as apathy, inertia, emotional numbness, and exhaustion. Depressed patients no longer feel creative or curious, and they often withdraw from their usual interests and hobbies.

Who wants to live only at a survival level? What are the current options you might be offered by your doctor if you appear to be depressed? Quite likely your physician or psychiatrist will prescribe an antidepressant, but don't let them fool you—in my experience with thousands of patients, pharmaceuticals are not a very good solution. In fact, they often worsen the situation!

Just How Depressing Are Antidepressants?

As a medical doctor, I of course believe that there are some medications that are necessary and helpful to patients when they have serious health conditions, but I'm here to tell you that antidepressant drugs are *not* on my good list! They are, in my opinion, among the most useless of all drugs.

It has been published in at least four major journals, including the esteemed *New England Journal of Medicine,* that if all studies were allowed to be published on the testing of antidepressant drugs, *both negative and positive,* the net results would be a big fat zero—no net benefit at all.

I know that this is a serious statement, but after treating more than 30,000 patients at the Shealy Pain Clinic who suffered from both pain and depression, I have to agree. I saw people walk into my office in a zombie-like state, tired and completely out of it, still anxious and depressed even though they had been prescribed antidepressants and antianxiety drugs by their doctor or psychiatrist—which is a ridiculous combination.

Rates of depression are not known with any accuracy, because so much is not reported or underreported. Some sources predict the rates are as high as 40 percent of Americans who are clinically depressed, which I personally do not doubt. The World Health Organization (WHO), in its report on mental illness released September 28, 2001, projected that depression will be the second largest killer after heart disease by 2020—and studies were already showing in 2001 that depression is a contributory factor to fatal coronary disease. These are pretty tragic and dismal statistics, but there is hope.

Personally, I think of depression as the foundation of a life that is majorly unfulfilled. Here is how I have arrived at this conclusion: Depression is one of the leading causes of disability, and it significantly contributes to many other very serious medical conditions, such as cancer and heart disease. Depressed people exhibit higher levels of cognitive decline and senility, while also struggling with weakness in their immune mechanisms and sluggish hormones.

It also speeds up all the aging processes to which our bodies are susceptible. I inevitably saw all these devastating conditions in my clinic among the sad and despondent patients who came to us.

The stages of descent into depression consist of an accumulation of melancholy moods, leading to a sense of being disconnected from one's inner joy or core values. These individuals found that they were unable to relate to the subtle sides of life, and they often could not control or stop their negative thoughts and feelings. This leads to imbalances in the nervous system and hormones, and eventually long-term chronic depression if nothing is done to try to reverse the decline.

I propose that the real causes of depression (and these are things that we can fix in ourselves) are many and varied. It sneaks in when we selectively focus on the worst aspects of our past, future, or daily experiences, and when we continue to fuss obsessively about what is wrong, missing, or unfair in our life. Allowing a habit of self-pity and absorption in our own frustrations keeps us stuck and makes things worse over time, eventually leading to feelings of alienation and cynicism.

Depression as a Downward Spiral

Things go from bad to worse when a depressed person converts a discouraging experience into a failure story by agonizing about it or perhaps deciding that it was their own fault due to weakness or lack of skill. More often than not, the individual then concludes that this must be a permanent weakness of character within him- or herself.

As I watched patients continue to feel more hopelessness and helplessness in their depression, they often began to blame others and external situations for the mental and emotional states that were developing. This interpretation is seriously flawed, in that it puts the center of power (to change and heal) outside of themselves—effectively disabling their natural ability to heal.

I believe that the cure for depression, and very often chronic pain, can be found when we learn to attune ourselves and dwell in the love and joy of our spiritual heart. From an inner place of peace and healing, we can use our own power and conscientiousness to dissolve negative beliefs and find the strength to accept our difficulties gracefully and patiently.

But I also saw that some days these individuals just could not rise above their depression, because they felt too hopeless and exhausted even to get up out of bed, let alone begin to eat better, exercise, and practice other healthy habits. Even saying the word *conscientiousness* would be too much for some of them on a bad day!

But through the Shealy Pain Clinic, we developed therapies and protocols that were incredibly successful in getting these people out of bed and out of their own way, as we guided them toward the path to wholeness.

But before getting into that, I'd like to step back and talk about my own early years just for a bit, so you can understand how I came to create these paths to health that so many have walked along. I was sympathetic by nature to their plight, through my own conscientiousness, but also because I experienced my own levels of pain along the way.

Experiencing Chronic Pain Firsthand

I've always been quite a healthy person who is seldom ill, but I know what it's like to struggle with pain. As a young adult, I was at a picnic at a local lake during the last weekend of my internship at Duke University. A group of us from the internal medicine internship program were just horsing around, climbing up on one another's shoulders and jumping off into the water. It was all innocent fun, but during the last climb, one of my fellow interns happened to put both feet on my right shoulder and jump. As he did, I got a sharp pain above my right shoulder.

That was the beginning of a long saga of neck problems that has plagued me in this life. During the next couple of years, I had intermittent pain, which was greatly aggravated whenever I over-used my right arm (as when lifting weights).

When it happened, my father recommended that I try his Electreat, an antique electrical stimulator that had helped him re-cover from a painful facial paralysis called Bell's palsy. During my entire career, I have seen only two other patients who had this painful condition; it is almost always painless. But in my father's case, physicians were unable to help his facial pain, so a chiroprac-tor gave him the Electreat, which helped him immensely.

I also tried it, but found it cumbersome and especially difficult to use for my neck pain. So I packed it away, not knowing at the time that this old relic would provide inspiration and direction later in my career.

A few years later, in the early 1960s, after my neurosurgery residency at Massachusetts General Hospital, we moved to Cleve-land, Ohio, where I joined the faculty at Western Reserve Hospi-tal. I knew I had to stay long enough to practice a minimum of two years before I could take the neurosurgical board exams. So I buckled down at Western Reserve, where I gained excellent clini-cal experience and a strong foundation in research.

This was an intense time of new learning for me, because the field of pain management was so badly in need of a fresh approach. You see, since the 1920s neurosurgeons had only two main ways of controlling pain: They would either cut the front half of the spinal cord, called a *cordotomy,* or destroy the most crucial part of personality by removing the frontal lobe in the brain, which was called a *lobotomy.* Both of these methods were horribly damaging and yielded more side effects than most drugs. And many of the drugs at that time were also brutal and debilitating.

I felt there must be better ways to control pain, and so did many other new thinkers, including the junior neurosurgeon at Western Reserve, Bill Collins, who, like me, was a very research-oriented person. Bill had developed an animal model for evaluating pain physiology in cats, and I was fortunate to have his model to explore.

Unfortunately, soon after I arrived, Bill could see there was someone competent to take over for him (namely me), so he left—first to become chair at the Medical College of Virginia, and then later at Yale. He told me that he had stayed 12 years in Cleveland until someone else came along! At his going-away party, I gave him the old Electreat as a joke. After all, the claims made back in 1919 about this thing seemed ridiculous—but that just shows you what I didn't know at the time!

My Early Research Forays into the World of Pain

While at Western Reserve, I obtained a grant from the National Institutes of Health (NIH) to do pain research, and over the next three years I produced some of my most important research. The essence of my work was to explore in-depth the anatomy and physiology of pain and look for nondestructive ways to control it.

Among other findings, I learned that most chronic pain travels primarily in the smallest C fibers in the body. About 60 percent of the C-fiber input crosses to the opposite side from the nerve, but 40 percent goes up the spinal cord on the same side as the incoming nerve. This explained to me why the results of a cordotomy seemed to last only a few years at most, if the operation worked at all.

I also discovered that the C-fiber activity disperses up and down the spinal cord for at least a few centimeters, which meant that the interconnections and alternative pathways are virtually unlimited for those pain messages to get to the brain. Through these findings, by the fall of 1964 I had a model for studying pain and began to evaluate physiological ways to suppress it.

Later the next year, I traveled to Canada to learn transsphenoidal hypophysectomy from Dr. Jules Hardy. I introduced that approach in the United States in 1965, and continued with it until I gave up surgery in 1974. However, I bring this up because, just before I left Reserve, I was doing this procedure, and as usual I was wearing a headlight to see deep into the wound. A nurse tripped over my headlight cord, pulling me back and sending me crashing to the floor. This was yet another accident that caused me many more years of neck and shoulder pain.

My research continued unabated, however, and I was in touch a few times about our work in pain physiology with Dr. Pat Wall, who was a well-known British neurophysiologist who worked at the Massachusetts Institute of Technology (MIT) back then. In the summer of 1965, Pat sent me a prepublication copy of his paper, "The Gate Control Theory of Pain." In the early fall of that year, I went to Boston to meet with Pat and discuss the implications. As I left his office, I said to Chardy, "If Pat is correct, we ought to be able to control pain by stimulating the dorsal columns of the spinal cord."

When I got back to Western Reserve, I mentioned my idea to the chair of neurosurgery and he replied, "My God, Norm, you have some wild ideas." Wild or not, my most important work at Western Reserve followed, and by the spring of 1966, I had proven beyond any reasonable doubt that stimulation of the dorsal columns, the back part of the spinal cord, could indeed inhibit pain. I was able to do this electrophysiologically, and also proved the same thing by implanting stimulators in cats that I could then test in an awake state after that implantation.

As soon as I passed my board exams, I bid Western Reserve Medical School good-bye. It had been three and a half years of tough work. As a family, we decided to move to Wisconsin for an opportunity that was too good to pass up.

Continuing My Work in Wisconsin

My new position was as chief of neurosciences at the Gundersen Clinic (now Gundersen Health System), one of the ten largest clinics in the U.S., and I held that post from 1966 to 1971. When I first arrived at Gundersen, I explained to them that my research grant at Western Reserve could not transfer, even though it still had two years to go. I reapplied for the same grant and was turned down; however, thanks to contacts by the Gundersen family, I did receive grants from the Boothroyd Foundation and was able to continue my research directions.

At first, I mainly continued chronic-pain work in animals with implanted dorsal column stimulators, such as I had been doing at Western Reserve. By the time I was ready to test my findings on human subjects, the animals had been stimulated for at least 18 months with no problems and no damage to the spinal cord.

So I approached an old friend, Tom Mortimer, whom I knew from my days at Western Reserve. Tom was a medical-engineering student who was working on his doctorate at the time, and I encouraged him to help me develop equipment that I could implant and test in humans to see if we could get the same results in dorsal column stimulation (DCS). I remembered the old Electreat technology and managed to get a second old device from the original manufacturer so I could show patients how electrical stimulation would feel.

Tom was able to make me a stimulator that could be implanted into humans, and in the spring of 1967 I found a patient willing to try it. I carefully explained to this man and his family that this procedure was experimental, but since the elderly gentleman had advanced cancer of the lung and was in a great deal of chest pain, he and his family all agreed that it would be worth a try.

So I implanted the stimulator Tom made, and the patient's pain was completely controlled. He did suffer a stroke ten days later due to complications from the cancer and died, but the autopsy showed that his spinal cord was normal.

The second subject, Ruth, came to my attention in October 1967 when one of the Gundersen surgeons asked me to evaluate a patient. She had cancer of the uterus and had been operated on several times and given all the radiation she was allowed, but still had significant pain. A psychiatrist consultant and I explained to her that with DCS we would be treating only her pain, not her cancer. She signed an informed consent, and I implanted a second individual with the DCS made by Tom Mortimer, who came up for the procedure. (At that point he had completed his doctorate, and he later went on to become an expert in muscle stimulation.)

This woman's pain was totally controlled in the first days after surgery. On the ninth day, I went in to get her ready to go home and found her in tears. "What use is it to be rid of my pain if I still have cancer?" she asked as she cried. I explained that we discussed before surgery that we were treating only her pain.

Ruth was a widow and had one son, who lived about 70 miles away. She lived seven years after the DCS implant. Always, when she was not depressed, her pain was well controlled. But when she became significantly depressed, her discomfort level was not well maintained, even with the DCS! This was something that I would see again and again in my life—the connection between pain and depression.

Pioneering Therapies for Pain and Depression

These first two successful cases were huge breakthroughs, and they led to two incredible innovations in pain management for humans: dorsal column stimulation and transcutaneous electrical nerve stimulation (TENS).

The dorsal column stimulator (DCS) that I pioneered is a surgically implanted device that uses small electrical currents from electrodes to adjust the electromagnetic fields within the spinal column. The stimulator was so successful in treating previously untreatable chronic back pain that it remains a treatment for pain by physicians worldwide.

TENS is the use of electrical current that's produced by a device to stimulate the skin nerves for therapeutic purposes. The unit is usually connected to the skin using two or more electrodes and can modulate pulse width, frequency, and intensity for the relief of pain and other symptoms. Likewise, the TENS system is also used everywhere to control pain, and while I don't personally hold the patent, I am considered the father of this technology. I went on to develop two of my own versions: the SheLi TENS (also called the Shealy PainPro) and GigaTENS, which were handheld devices that I used extensively in my practice.

The Liss Cranial Electrical Stimulator (CES) is another device that I developed for treatment of depression. It is a small unit that puts out 15, 500, and 15,000 pulses per second, usually used at a strength of one to two milliamps. It is used on the right and left temples or on the back and front of the head, primarily to reduce depression and ease pain through increasing levels of serotonin and beta-endorphins.

When I developed the Shealy PainPro, I was able to prove that this device could relieve chronic pain in almost all subjects. It's used to simulate areas of pain, or to activate acupuncture points, for relief of discomfort. We knew it worked through clinical studies, and found out later that one reason why it works on both pain and depression is because it raises the patient's level of DHEA. I went on to patent this system, and it has been widely used today by traditional and nontraditional practitioners in nearly every specialty where a pain problem needs to be resolved.

I also developed the Shealy RelaxMate, a highly successful adjunct for relaxation. This device resembles glasses or goggles and works by flashing lights at a slow rate, which puts 90 percent of people into a deep state of relaxation within about five minutes. The idea for this product came to me from hearing that pulses of light used in radar monitoring in World War II were found to put people who watched them into a trance.

Along the way, I also pioneered facet rhizotomy—a safe surgical procedure for back pain in which nerve fibers are destroyed by radio-frequency heat or phenol alcohol in order to reduce pain coming from the joints in the back. I also developed an advanced computerized traction table for treatment of headaches and back pain.

There Are Many Paths to Health and Wellness

But lest you feel that my discussion of the pursuit of health and wellness is all about devices and complicated medical procedures, there is so much more to it. There are very powerful techniques and therapies we've used very effectively in our pain clinic that you can use at home. I developed most of these after I went out on my own in 1971.

Leaving the Gundersen Clinic, where I was successful and salaried, to go into private practice was one of the most critical decisions of my professional life. People told me at the time how courageous it was to take this path, to move away from academic medicine and such a highly respected traditional clinical setting and go into (what was at that time!) the totally unknown world of "alternative medicine."

Of course, I simply did what appeared essential to me personally, which was to explore any direction where there was exciting potential. With that in mind—and with the blessings of my dear wife, who totally believed that I could do it—I opened The Pain Rehabilitation Center in October 1971. To my knowledge, that was the first use of the phrase "pain rehabilitation," but a lot of the time people still referred to us as the Shealy Pain Clinic.

From the beginning, I had more than enough patients to fill the 25-bed unit that I developed at St. Francis Hospital in La Crosse. But now I had to develop alternatives to offer those pain patients who were not candidates for DCS. Many of the protocols we created for them were related to behavior modification and self-regulation, and these approaches worked extremely well.

To begin with, we knew that physical activity was absolutely critical to helping people with pain and depression get back into the swing of life. So I set up a program where patients were out of bed at 7 A.M. and not allowed to go back to bed until 9 P.M. Five days a week, they went to the YMCA for an hour of water aerobics. They were assigned tasks such as walking the hall so many lengths a day and going to physical therapy. This regime was a huge wake-up call for most of them, who had become accustomed to lying down all day in misery and pain.

We carefully monitored their diets and made sure they were eating nutritious food, staying away from junk food, soda pop, candy, and other bad habits that would zap their energy or affect their overall health in negative ways.

At one point, I asked a young psychiatrist for assistance and he suggested, "Why don't we try group therapy three times a week?" I agreed, but with the caveat that there was to be no bitching and moaning during the sessions. When I found out later that these group sessions had become nothing more than a place to complain, I quickly sent the young psychiatrist packing.

I continued using the electro-acupuncture therapy techniques that I had pioneered and used since the mid-60s, whereby we put needles into the center of the patient's pain, with a second and third needle above and below the sensitive area. We stimulated these needles electrically, so that the subject would know how electrical stimulation felt. In addition, all patients were treated with the Electreat at least twice daily.

Two to four times a day, nurses went around to each person and gave vigorous slapping massages around and on the pain areas. Tongue depressors were also frozen into paper cups and acted as Popsicles to use for massaging areas of pain to desensitize them.

At this time, I also introduced a drug-withdrawal technique that had been pioneered by Dr. Wilbert E. Fordyce. Dr. Fordyce was a psychologist at the University of Washington in Seattle who worked with chronic-pain patients through behavioral modification, too. Following his lead, we gradually diluted the patients' medication in cocoa syrup, giving them a little bit less each day. I instructed the nurses to ignore all complaints of pain or pain behavior. I made rounds daily, and patients knew they were not allowed to talk about their pain unless specifically asked.

Introducing the Power of Relaxation

In the fall of 1973, at the urging of a friend, I took the Silva Method class. During two weekends, I spent ten or more hours, for a total of four days, relaxing and experiencing just good old early-20th-century self-hypnosis. It is one thing to read about self-regulation, but it is quite different to experience it for yourself. At the end of those four days, I realized how much you can change your attitude and reduce stress by immersion into deep relaxation.

So early in 1974, I took this newfound experience and began a different approach to my intense work with chronic-pain patients. I reduced the number of weeks they spent in the behavioral-modification program from four weeks to only three. On the last three days of each program, I spent eight hours daily meeting with all patients, taking them through relaxation exercises, guided imagery, and related self-hypnosis techniques.

At that time, I did not know enough different mental exercises to last for 24 hours, but I did have lots of books. So I would take the patients down to the gym, and the ones who could lie down would do so on the mats while I led them through guided-imagery meditations and other self-regulation exercises from my stack of books.

When we incorporated this approach, our data showed an increase from the usual 75 percent success rate to more than 80 percent in only three weeks! That's more than 5 percent higher in a program that was one week shorter than it had been before. We amazed even ourselves.

That year, I also experienced one of the most dramatic events of my clinical life. On April 30, a 50-year-old woman whom I will call Abby arrived by air ambulance to us. She was quite ill, suffering with widespread metastatic breast cancer, unable to walk, and hardly able to eat or drink. Throughout the first two weeks of our modification program, she kept insisting, "I did not come here to be brainwashed. I came to get rid of my pain."

I repeatedly told her, "If you would just shut up and listen, I am teaching you how to get rid of your pain." Just over two weeks later, on May 17, something amazing happened. Abby was brought in by stretcher and moved to a mat on the floor. At midmorning I took the group through a 20-minute exercise by Roy Masters on forgiveness with repeated subliminal messages to reinforce forgiveness.

There were 53 other patients with her in the room also experiencing the same exercise. When I finished, Abby was still lying on the floor in a deep trance—the first time this had ever happened for her or anyone in my classes! She did not come back to normal awareness as the others had and lay there repetitively moving her arms up and down, deeply unaware of anything else.

I went over, congratulated her on being so deep, and counted her up to normal consciousness. Abby smiled, got up, and walked out of the room—*pain free!* To me, it was just like a scene from Our Lady of Lourdes shrine in France, a place of sacred healing where miracles are said to occur. She then flew home on a commercial plane.

The lesson she taught me was very clear: I knew then that behavior and function could be controlled far better by mental self-regulation than simple operant conditioning (behavior modification).

Transform Your Life Through Autogenic Training

If you take nothing else from these lessons, please know that practicing self-regulation each day for about 20 minutes is a tremendous factor in securing a healthy future for yourself. This kind of routine comes naturally to many conscientious people, who see and feel the difference immediately upon trying it and know how important it is to make time for it each day as part of their health regime.

Since I first learned about it almost 40 years ago, I have personally done autogenic training (AT) daily, since it is my preferred and recommended form of self-regulation. I could see right away that it had tremendous potential to help the patients who were under our care at the Shealy Pain Clinic, and, as I just discussed, we built this kind of therapy into their routine.

Autogenic training is a series of statements that you repeat slowly to yourself while breathing deeply, similar to a guided meditation. You gradually reinforce messages to your body and mind that all is well, and it promotes a sublime feeling of relaxation and serenity. I feel that this particular approach to self-regulation, which was originally developed by J. H. Schultz, has the greatest level of scientific proof of efficacy than any other meditation or self-regulation technique in the world today.

More than 50 years after Schultz first introduced his autogenic training method, six full volumes were published on it with an astonishing 2,600 scientific references. That's even before it became part of autogenic-feedback training, and later biofeedback!

Doing autogenic training at home is easy. Each of the following six statements takes only three minutes each, so within 18 minutes you can feel a deep sense of calm:

You start with assuming a comfortable position. I find that a reclining chair is ideal. Close your eyes, and as you breathe in, say this slowly to yourself: "My arms and legs . . ."; as you breathe out, finish the thought: ". . . are heavy and warm." As you do this, imagine the sun beaming down upon your arms and legs. Do this for three minutes daily for one week.

In the second week, after the three minutes described above, repeat the exercise, but this time add on these two phrases: "My heartbeat is . . . calm and regular." Continue for three minutes, while visualizing something calm and regular, such as the pendulum of a clock.

Each of the next four weeks, increase by another three minutes, adding one more set of phrases: "My breathing is . . . free and easy" (visualizing something free and easy, such as a bird gliding through the air without having to flap its wings); "My abdomen . . . is warm" (visualizing the sun beaming down upon your abdomen); "My forehead . . . is cool" (visualizing yourself outside, warmly dressed, with a cool breeze blowing across your forehead); and finally, "My mind . . . is quiet and still" (visualizing a pleasant, quiet, still scene). By the end of the sixth week, you will have a full, very powerful 18-minute exercise.

Once you have down the basic autogenic training technique, then you can add organ-specific phrases if you have a precise need within your body. Just remember to use only positive phrases and images. So for habits such as smoking, use "I am free . . . of smoking," or use "My weight is . . . ideal for me" for body-image issues. You could do this while visualizing yourself on scales in front of a mirror, seeing your body at your ideal weight. This practice retrains your brain, your nervous system, and your body's autonomic control system.

The Biogenics Route to Self-Regulation

There are many versions of similar exercises that train the body and mind to relax deeply and rebalance. Biogenics is the program I developed that is somewhat like the AT method but customized as per my own research. It is made up of a series of more than 30 different CDs I recorded with my voice that you can use to retrain your central nervous system. Listening to these CDs helps you calm down; break down blocks; stop unhealthy habits; and get back to normal, healthy functioning.

I based Biogenics on the research that I completed through my Ph.D. studies, which were taken in humanistic psychology at Saybrook Institute in California (now called Saybrook University). When I graduated in 1977, this was the leading school in this field in the country, and it is still active today.

From that experience and research, I created a workbook for self-regulation training to be used by instructors. It was essentially a software program for biofeedback training, and this content also became my best-selling book called *90 Days to Self-Health.*

Between 1977 and 1979, *90 Days to Self-Health* sold 130,000 copies (30,000 in hardcover and 100,000 in paperback). For many years to follow, I regularly led a five-day workshop for health professionals on Biogenics, the trademarked name I gave to my self-regulation program.

How Autogenic Training Improves Conscientiousness

When we introduced these mental exercises to patients who were suffering from pain and depression, we saw tremendous progress, as presented earlier. But anyone can benefit from them, even children as young as five years old. Athletes, students, businesspeople, and patients of all kinds can improve their health and longevity when they apply these simple techniques. It is said that 80 percent of stress illnesses can be managed with just autogenic training, and I certainly believe that.

For example, in the 1970s I taught this technique to the football team at the University of Wisconsin–La Crosse. They had been at the bottom of their league the year before, but they became co-champions of the league the season they started AT.

The girls' basketball team at the same university used a specific autogenic recording of a guided imagery that I made for them. Half the team just practiced; the other half used the self-regulation recording. The players who listened to the recording were 80 percent more successful at free throws than those who did not.

In a more recent study of the effectiveness of an herbal preparation on hypertension, 30 percent of the patients failed to improve with the herb. However, autogenic training brought the blood pressure of 12 of the 14 patients down to normal within ten minutes, and those patients continued to have improved blood pressure readings at their follow-up appointments.

Within six months of practicing autogenic training techniques daily in a conscientious manner, many people begin to see spiritual imagery within their mind's eye, leading to spontaneous meditation and contact with the Divine. And that is where my story is going next. There is so much more out there than we usually see on this earth, so much potential wisdom to learn and guidance for you to tap into.

I believe that my own metaphysical journey is one you can take, too—anyone can, and many do! Come along with me, and open your mind to a world of infinite possibilities and a long, conscientious, and peaceful life.

∽∽∽ ∽∽∽

CHAPTER FIVE

TAPPING INTO
THE KNOWLEDGE
OF THE AGES

Those of you who were around in 1972 likely remember what you were doing that summer. Change was in the air, and traditional belief systems were being challenged at all levels of society. The government was taxing us into the ground, while at the same time desperately trying to reassert its control. The politicians did not know the extent of the profound societal changes that were coming—nor did they embrace them.

But I did. I embraced the newness of ideas. I was right in the middle of it—along with the other free thinkers—and to us, the possibilities seemed endless. I remember believing that I could change the world, get the medical system back on track, and get the government off our backs. My family was young, my career was going very well, my research efforts were paying off, and I saw no reason not to explore everything this world had to offer.

It all sounds quite simple, but this was a pretty big leap. Up to this point, I was a relatively straightforward thinking, scientific-based neurosurgeon. But suddenly I started hearing about so many other therapies and spiritual ideas out there—about colonics, auras, crystals, different chiropractic approaches, balancing chakras, autogenic training, past-life therapy, and so many other emerging concepts—and I just wanted to know more and more.

As I've explained, I was very concerned that the traditional medical approaches, which were based primarily on offering medication or discussing surgery options, were not really helping the patients who were coming to the clinic. I was seeing the ones who

53

no one else could seem to help. I was propelled forward by my own conscientious drive to do good for them, to find better solutions that would relieve them of their pain and depression.

There wasn't really any way to tell at the time where all this would take me, but before long I became the founder and first president of the American Holistic Medical Association (AHMA). Through meetings across the country, I found myself aligned with an incredible group of like-minded individuals by the mid-1970s, and we all agreed to seek the possibility of establishing the AHMA. There was just so much information and misinformation out there on holistic medicine and alternative therapies as related to medical care, that I knew the time was right to put a credible organization in place so that we could keep advancing and refining the knowledge.

So when we sat down together, we easily compiled a total of about 3,000 physician names just from the contacts already present in the room. Over the next six months, I took the lead to organize a campaign to gather more supporters who might be interested in membership. Of course, the American Medical Association refused to allow our ads in any of its publications, so we just got the word out ourselves through the good old postal system, since this was well before the Internet!

And so it was in May 1978 that we held the founding meeting of the American Holistic Medical Association in Denver. We had 212 physicians and medical students present and spent several days developing a consensus on the bylaws and constitution. We also had an all-day scientific meeting and held elections for the first official board and officers.

Knowing that I already had a heavy patient load and an extensive travel schedule, I hoped someone else would be selected to serve as president. However, they elected me. At the end of the meeting, the members gave me what became one of my favorite bolo ties—a silver phoenix with turquoise representing the bird rising from ashes. I have always treasured this gift of the phoenix as a sign that we were starting something big—something that represented our tapping into true medical wisdom and spiritual healing—that would change the world.

Conscientious People Are Very Good at Causes

Maybe I was elected to that leadership role with the AHMA because the group that was assembled could see that Chardy and I were just the kind of conscientious individuals who would work night and day once we took something like this on. Well, they were right. We did work night and day. It didn't matter that I had a busy clinic and a full career on the go, or that Chardy was a full-time mother of three with her own community and professional interests, projects, and passions.

Notwithstanding any of this, we added the cause of holistic medicine to our plates and made it work. The other leaders of the AHMA movement did as much as they could, too; and as a collective, we were always planning something. Since it was the days before e-mail and social media, we addressed thousands of envelopes over the next few years, spoke on the phone all the time, and got together for conferences and group meetings as often as we could. The AHMA hosted professionals from around the world who would come to speak on their specialties, and they hosted me and others when we would travel abroad.

One place I always enjoyed visiting, and where I was always warmly received, was at the offices of the Association for Research and Enlightenment (A.R.E.) in Virginia Beach, Virginia. Chardy and I began attending their annual conferences starting in 1972, which began a lifelong association with the A.R.E. group that has been extremely valuable to me. The founder of the A.R.E. was Edgar Cayce, who is generally considered the father of holistic and energy medicine and arguably the most talented and prolific intuitive of the 20th century. I have researched and referred to his work extensively in many of my previous books.

So by around 1971, I had begun lecturing around the world on various topics—at medical schools, universities, hospitals, and churches—with up to 100 appearances each year. I think that by 1978 I was living the busiest year of my whole life! I spent 180 days out of town that year on scheduled workshops and lectures, and pretty well loved every minute of it. I was able to do it because Chardy had full control of things at home and supported me wholeheartedly. Likewise, my staff at the clinic knew the rehabilitative pain program inside out and kept things moving along seamlessly.

Along with my travels, I was often asked to speak on national TV programs, and so I appeared on *The Tomorrow Show, The Joan Rivers Show, Geraldo, Good Morning America, Today, The Oprah Winfrey Show,* the Wisdom Channel, and dozens of other regional and local television and radio programs.

I am retired from most of this today, but over the years I produced more than 325 publications on a wide range of traditional medical issues and alternative-medicine topics, including 29 books. I have no plans to stop publishing books, and I enjoy compiling and sending a free weekly newsletter that still goes out to thousands of subscribers. And for more than two decades I have hosted the most popular call-in radio show in the Ozarks here in Missouri on KWTO 560 AM. I plan to keep that up as well for as long as they'll have me. Each week, there are always more callers seeking advice, and now the program is streamed online so that anyone in the world can tune in on Thursday afternoons. And I do get calls from all over the country!

Tracing the Roots of My Own Conscientiousness

I firmly believe that one of the great gifts I received in this life was my parents. Even though they raised me to attend and follow the traditional teachings of the Methodist Church, they did not indoctrinate me with rigid religious beliefs that strangled creativity and free thought. I grew up with permission to explore fully the multidimensional reality of life on both the material and spiritual planes.

My mother herself would occasionally visit a psychic woman in our town, for example, so I grew up accepting the world of intuition. Lil Brown, as she was known, was accepted throughout the southeast as an excellent psychic; supposedly she had been consulted by the governor and other prominent figures. So it did not seem strange at all to me that certain people knew things that others did not, or that some individuals could foresee the future. But I also accepted that not everything a mystical person said was the God-given truth; for every respected intuitive, there appeared to be dozens of others who were complete flakes. (This isn't unlike the odds within the ranks of our current politicians, now that I think about it!)

Anyway, it was always entertaining to hear what Lil Brown had to say. Shortly before I left for college, my mother asked Lil to do a reading for me. She said, "You will become well known, but you will never be President of the United States." That was a relief! I can't imagine a worse profession than being a politician, although I have been said to have some of the same gifts, such as my ability and conviction to speak and be heard.

Even as a child, I was encouraged to develop my own point of view, and that's also where the roots of my inquisitiveness, conscientiousness, and openness to new ideas began. I stated out loud at age four that I would become a doctor, and no one was surprised; they encouraged me from that point on to excel in that direction and toward *any* goal I set for myself.

Since I was blessed with remarkably nurturing parents, who were themselves hardworking and conscientious souls, I always knew that my life had a purpose. I conscientiously followed that purpose, even though sometimes I was not absolutely clear where I was going.

Early in my own spiritual journey, I realized and accepted that each of us has a choice about what we come to this earthly life to learn. I believe that we choose the main people we will come in contact with in this realm, even before we're born, so that we can learn the right lessons and fulfill our purpose.

This means that whether your parents were good or bad, you chose them. Likewise, that boss who drives you crazy or the spouse who fully supports you—all your relationships, some seemingly bad and others good, were all chosen by you in order to learn. When you accept that each experience provides you with just the right challenges you need, you can accept that sometimes you have to deal with nasty individuals or face disappointing or tragic circumstances. It is the combination of all your experiences that helps you develop a stronger character and gives you the most appropriate abilities in order to achieve your life's purpose.

Discovering Energy Medicine

In my own life, it appeared that my purpose involved both the worlds of traditional and alternative medicine this time around. I chose to study the medical science route first, and practiced as a neurosurgeon and researcher for many years before my eyes became open to other modalities.

One of the first new ideas I embraced was energy medicine, specifically in the form of acupuncture. As a neuroscientist, I knew that everything we do in medicine involves some kind of energy, and I accepted from my training and experience that all body systems are interrelated. Therefore, when I read about acupuncture and the concept that the body has 12 main meridians through which our life energy flows, this made sense to me.

Essentially, these meridians represent vector potentials from the organs of the body. Energy runs from the organs out along the specific paths (the 12 meridians) to the tip of each meridian (at the tips of the toenails or fingernails, usually) and back. I understood how acupuncture had a way of completing the circuits through needles, tapping, or massage. In doing so, the practitioner could restore the natural functioning of the patient's vital organs, as well as improve their energy level and overall health. I enjoyed learning about acupuncture on my own for many years before finding ways to get more formal training.

Being the inquisitive person that I was, from the time I first started studying acupuncture I wondered what would happen if I introduced controlled electrical currents to these circuits or others in the body—an idea that was relatively new at the time. I did manage to perfect this technique and introduce it successfully in my clinic to help my patients overcome chronic pain, breaking new ground in this field.

A Western Form of Acupuncture

In January 1972, the *Wall Street Journal* featured an article about acupuncture. The American media jumped on what, for them, seemed to be a new and mysterious concept, because it had been used to treat *New York Times* journalist James Reston after an emergency appendectomy that he underwent while covering Richard Nixon's historic trip to China.

The newspaper article quoted Janet Travell, M.D., Kennedy's former physician and a leading expert in the field of myofascial pain, and she said, essentially, "What's all this fuss about acupuncture? There's a young neurosurgeon in Wisconsin who has a Western form of acupuncture."

She was referring to me, of course. I met Janet first in 1966. Shortly after the article came out, I received a letter from Dr. Paul Dudley White, Eisenhower's former physician and one of the first physicians to visit China after the thaw in tensions between the two countries.

Dr. White heard about my concept of Western acupuncture and asked me to visit him. In April, I flew to Boston to see this highly esteemed man, the grand Brahman of Boston medicine. At 84 years old, he had just flown back from Europe that day and was seeing patients. He spent a lively two hours discussing my work with me and how it related to acupuncture.

A month later, I received a phone call out of the blue. "I am Bob Matson, president of the Academy of Parapsychology and Medicine," the man began. "We are holding a symposium on acupuncture in June at Stanford University. Dr. Paul Dudley White is to speak, and he said you know much more about acupuncture than he does. Would you replace him on the program?" Who could refuse that?

So in June of 1972, I flew to San Francisco for the meeting, and that was one of the events that changed my life forever. I presented a paper entitled "A Physiological Basis for Electro-Acupuncture." Having some right suprascapular pain myself, I volunteered to have Dr. Felix Mann, a British physician who had practiced acupuncture in London for 11 years, work on my neck and shoulder. The session was filmed live for the 1,200 attending physicians.

While this was all very exciting to be part of, from my point of view the most critical aspect of this whole conference was meeting so many other highly respected healing professionals for the first time. In addition to meeting Felix, I also met Dr. William Tiller, who was a leading materials scientist interested in parapsychology. I met Drs. Gladys and Bill McGarey of the A.R.E. Clinic in Phoenix. Dr. Phil Toyama was also there; he was a Japanese American physician and acupuncturist, and I enjoyed getting to know him.

It was a particular honor to meet renowned spiritual healer Olga Worrall of Baltimore. All of them, especially Olga, went on to become lifelong friends and colleagues of mine—and fellow supporters of the AHMA cause.

A year later, during a trip to London in 1973, I arranged to take a one-week acupuncture course with Dr. Felix Mann. Felix had one of the largest white-energy auras I have ever seen around anyone, but I could not get him to discuss anything metaphysical. Despite his tight lips, he helped refine my use of acupuncture, which I had begun in the mid-1960s.

Incidentally, also in 1973, I met with one of the first delegations of Chinese physicians who came to visit the U.S. after the thaw in relations between the two countries. They had heard about my work with electrical therapy and asked to visit my clinic. In fact, they had started using electrical stimulation of acupuncture needles at the same time I did!

An Awakening of Medical Intuition

Around this same time, I became very interested in medical intuition. In December 1972, I flew to Chicago to meet Henry Rucker, a charismatic and highly intuitive person I had felt guided to meet. As I walked in for the one-hour appointment we had made, Henry said, "I've been waiting ten years for you. My teacher told me you would come."

Our appointment ended up lasting three hours, and he knew more about me than I did about myself! I was impressed enough to invite him back to La Crosse, Wisconsin, so I could find out more about his gifts as a medical intuitive. I wanted to see how effective he would be in making medical diagnoses in a clinical setting dealing with patients.

So it was in January 1973 that Henry arrived in La Crosse along with seven other psychic friends. They were part of the Psychic Research Foundation of Chicago, and all of them were keen to see if they had the talents I was talking about related to psychic diagnosis.

I had asked my 25 patients whether they would be interested in working with this group from Chicago and having a psychic diagnosis done. They all agreed. One at a time, the patients entered my office. Then Henry and his psychic friends each wrote down their impressions of the patient without asking a thing.

Henry himself was 70 percent accurate, and, when everyone in the group agreed on a diagnosis, they were 98 percent accurate. The results were impressive, and I knew I wanted to work more closely with Henry. I wanted him to counsel my patients, essentially to become a pastoral counselor at my clinic that was housed within St. Francis Hospital in La Crosse.

Henry had founded a metaphysical church called something along the lines of The Church of the Holy Light of Hermetic Wisdom, and I told him I was concerned that the name of his church would not work. As we explored other names, I thought about the name "Science of Mind," which I had recently discovered. No trademark or national registration of that name existed, so Henry and I founded The Science of Mind Church of Chicago. Henry was introduced as a pastoral counselor at my clinic, and before long, his reputation as a phenomenal counselor spread rapidly. A good number of area nurses, physicians, and even other clergymen sought consultations with him.

For example, our minister asked to see Henry because his 16-year-old son had a terrible problem with drugs. In fact, the young man was incarcerated at a reform school in Florida. Henry heard about the case and reassured the family, "Don't worry. He will be home soon."

The following day, the son phoned his parents and requested that he be allowed to come home. He had escaped from reform school. His parents agreed to take him back, but under the condition that he attend a counseling session in Chicago with Henry. The boy walked out of that session and asked, "Why didn't anyone ever talk to me like that before?!"

After that, the son never touched drugs again and has had a successful life for these past 40 years. One hour with Henry was better than years of conventional psychotherapy. He was, without question, the best one-on-one therapist I have ever known. He had a sense of what was wrong with a person, not only physically but also spiritually, and I saw how his unique form of intuitive counseling helped patients overcome mental and physical illnesses, addictions, and chronic pain of many kinds.

The year after meeting Henry, I came across another medical intuitive who also had tremendous accuracy. His name was Dr. Robert Leichtman, a board-certified internist by training. When I tested Bob, he was 96 percent accurate as a medical intuitive on making psychological diagnoses, but only 80 percent accurate on physical diagnoses. He said that was because he trained himself to "visit the mind." Very often, he would write three to five pages describing in great detail the individual's personality traits, both good and not so good. Like so many of these fine people whom I met over the years, Bob and I became lifelong colleagues in this field.

Working with Past-Life Regression Therapy

In the early 1970s, I found out that many alternative thera-pists used a type of treatment called past-life therapy (PLT) as a way to help clients overcome some mental, physical, or spiritual block that they might be facing that was causing them grief in this lifetime.

Many answers would arise through this therapy, which in-volved being hypnotized or placed in a state of reverie and then taken on a guided tour of previous experiences in this life that they may have blocked or returned to memories of previous life-times—memories that are stored in our souls. Some people easi-ly visit their past lives when guided to do so through therapy or meditation, but a smaller percentage find it hard to reach back and visit these experiences. I expect, perhaps, that some people just aren't ready to face those memories, or there is simply no need for them to do so at that time.

But as for myself, I have come to learn of dozens of specific past lives that my soul has lived in centuries gone by. I feel that learning of these experiences did lead me to a greater level of un-derstanding of my own path this time around—specifically, why certain things have happened to me and why I am the way I am.

One of the first past-life therapists who worked with me told me that I was trying to cram seven lifetimes into one! Another time, a woman gave me a past-life reading that seemed amazingly real to me. She said my neck problems in this life were related to a life I had lived in the ancient Middle East as a leader of a small Jewish tribe. I led the tribe into war against another tribe, but we were defeated. I spent the rest of that life in a yoke working like an ox, which certainly explained some of the chronic-pain episodes I suffered with at various times in this life.

In the fall of 1972, I met with a small group of friends once a week for PLT sessions, and we took turns guiding one anoth-er to visit past lives that lived on in our subconscious memories. On one occasion, I suggested that we try to progress into the fu-ture rather than the past. My friend Gary led the session, during which I saw myself living southwest of La Crosse and riding horses across rolling hills with my wife, Chardy. In the distance, I saw a white building, which I knew was related to the future of medicine somehow. This was pure precognition—because I did end up building a medical-research center on our ranch in Missouri 30 years later. And that building is now a home for the future of conscientious psychology!

In my opinion, the premier past-life therapist today is a man named Dr. Morris Netherton, who teaches and certifies past-life therapists in a two-part, three-week program at Holos Institutes of Health Inc.

Discovering the Mesmerizing Dr. John Elliotson

My most recent past-life experience is the one life that I feel most strongly to be true. It came to my conscious mind in January 1973. I had traveled to Aspen, Colorado, for a meeting of the Neuroelectric Society and was sitting in the audience at the time.

Just before my talk, Dr. William S. Kroger, a specialist in obstetrics, gynecology, and endocrinology and an expert in hypnosis, tried to convince us that acupuncture *was* hypnosis. I sat there strongly disagreeing, figuring he was full of crap, when he said, ". . . and, in the last century, there was a British physician who demonstrated that you could operate on mesmerized patients. His name was John Elliotson." (A mesmerized patient would be one who was under hypnosis.)

At the mere mention of John Elliotson's name, I felt as if someone rubbed a big piece of ice down my spine. I thought, *My God, I was John.* I just *knew* that this was true—the feeling was so strong. After the talk, I asked Bill for more information, but he knew little else. Prior to that evening, I felt neutral about the concept of reincarnation; however, at that moment, I suddenly felt absolutely certain. I *was* the reincarnation of this doctor who lived 100 years before, and I wanted to find out more.

When I returned home, I asked our hospital medical librarian to find more information about Dr. John Elliotson, but she found nothing. So I flew to London to find out for myself.

Upon touching down at Heathrow Airport, I got into a cab and said, "Take me to the Royal College of Surgeons," because I figured that they would have records of this man. But as the cab turned right, I was lifted off the backseat (quite literally!), and I felt that icy feeling go down my spine again. I knew we had to go in the opposite direction, and I gave the driver instructions suddenly to turn around and head the other way.

Sure enough, I found a small, round, brick building. I got out of the cab and went over to it. Once inside, I knew I had been there before. I somehow recognized every room, even though I had never visited anywhere near this place in my lifetime as Norm Shealy! But I knew each corridor intimately, because it was the place where John Elliotson had worked.

I then decided to visit the Royal College of Physicians to re-search his background further, and I confirmed that Elliotson had been born in 1795 and died in 1868. He was a British physician who introduced *mesmerism* (the early name for hypnosis) into England, and he had indeed worked in that same building I had just discovered.

Two Men, Two Different Lifetimes, but a Shared Existence

While in England, I went on to learn a great deal more about John, and there were so many striking similarities between his life and career path and my own life this time around, that I became truly convinced that I was the reincarnation of this man.

For example, Elliotson had a limp from childhood. At age nine, I was told I would have a limp forever, but instead I overcame it. Elliotson had striking black curly hair. As a young child, I desperately wanted black hair; I always hated my own blond hair. At about age five, I snuck up behind an aunt of mine who had black curly hair and cut off a lock. At age 16, just as I prepared for college, I asked my mother to dye my hair black so I could finally feel normal. While I loved that look at the time, I didn't keep my hair black, as it was too much trouble to maintain.

Elliotson was the first physician in London to give up wearing knickers and high socks. At age nine, I refused to wear knickers, and my mother and I had more than one battle royal about it. She could not understand it, but I stood my ground—I would not wear them, and she couldn't make me. In school, Elliotson was a Latin scholar, and so was I. In fact, I found the language easy to master compared to many of my school-age peers who hated learning it.

I found out that, like me, Elliotson was a medical pioneer in the field of pain management; he was the one who introduced narcotics to the medical world in London as a new form of controlling pain. In this life, my passion has been to get patients *off* their dependence on narcotics and find other ways to manage their pain.

In the academic world, Elliotson was the first professor of medicine at the University College London Hospital. Even though I was going into neurosurgery, I interned in medicine. He also introduced the stethoscope in London; I think perhaps that this is why I felt attracted to the field of internal medicine.

Elliotson introduced mesmerism in London. I began doing hypnotherapy and PLT sessions with no formal training, because it came completely naturally to me. Elliotson demonstrated that mesmerized patients, those under hypnosis, could make medical diagnoses, and I'd begun working with medical intuitives before I ever heard his name or knew anything about his work in this field.

Covering Even More Common Ground

Furthermore, Elliotson had made a reputation for himself as a physician who gave lectures to the public. Since 1971, I have done far more lecturing to the public than to physicians, that is for sure. And even more of a coincidence, Elliotson left academic medicine because of opposition he felt to his public demonstration of mesmerism; no one would accept this new therapy as having any validity. Six months earlier in my life, before I knew anything about this man, I had written an anonymous novel on the hypocrisy of medicine with regard to accepting new ideas. It was always a bugaboo of mine, and I'd left medical academia because of bureaucracy!

As I explored John's work further, I came upon his Harverian lecture given 130 years earlier on exactly the same topic, and it used many of the same examples that I did in 1972!

I count this experience of discovering my connection to Dr. Elliotson as the beginning of a major philosophical awakening in my life. This was proof positive to me that not only do we reincarnate, but we often carry with us many traits, beliefs, and values from previous lives. With all that John accomplished, I knew that he had to have been a highly conscientious person. I feel that many of my personality traits and my conscientious nature come from the influence of having been him in a past life.

Over the years since the point that I spontaneously "knew" that I was John, I have consulted with more than 100 psychics and intuitives about my experiences, and they all agree that I was indeed John.

Benefits of Past-Life Regression Therapy to Resolve Pain and Depression

My story of John's life and my relation to it can also be read in Walter Semkiw, M.D.'s, *Return of the Revolutionaries*. By the time this book came out, I had experienced many other spontaneous recalls and at least 20 guided PLT sessions where I gained more insights about my current life. Many of my spontaneously revealed incarnations have been confirmed by one or more talented intuitives.

As a result, I have also conducted hundreds of successful PLT sessions with patients, friends, family members, and students. *This is the most powerful psychotherapeutic tool available to us.* As Denys Kelsey said to me when I was fortunate enough to have a session with him, "Twelve hours on my couch will equal 18 months of the best conventional psychotherapy."

I consider Kelsey the patriarch of PLT, and I wholeheartedly agree with him. In fact, I'll even take it one step further: A single PLT session can be better than *18 years* of conventional psychotherapy! I no longer "believe" in reincarnation; I *know* that this is the reality in which we live.

That is why in 1972, shortly after I began adding autogenic training to the daily activities of my patients, I also began doing PLT sessions with those who seemed to have the greatest blocks to overcome. The power to heal that we were able to access in a clinical setting using this therapy was incredible. I helped patients uncover many fascinating stories that facilitated their healing over the years, but one of the very first cases is a good example of the benefit of this kind of therapy, so I will recount it here.

At the time, I was treating a young woman with intractable pain and paraplegia (paralysis) following a gunshot wound through her abdomen and spine. For the sake of privacy, let me simply call her Lela. She told me upon admission to the clinic that she had shot herself accidentally while cleaning her husband's gun. He was a policeman, so this sounded plausible.

However, when I did a PLT session with her, she recalled a remarkable story that sounded like the account of Anne Boleyn's life, right up to the rolling of her head after the guillotine. Lela faced and went through death in this experience that she revisited.

Afterward I asked her, "Lela, what does this mean?"

She was amnesic for an entire hour, unable to remember the details. Fortunately, I had recorded the session and was able to play it back to her with her permission. Then I asked the question again. This time she replied, "I don't know. The last thing I remember is that my husband and I were arguing. I was told when I awoke after surgery that I shot myself accidentally while cleaning his gun."

She had just revisited a life where she had died as a martyred wife, and I could see this revelation as a form of allegory. I replied to her, "I know. You think your husband shot you." Then she broke into tears, able to face the reality of her situation, which is the first step in healing.

Indeed, it's never possible to know whether the past life that was revealed to her actually happened at some earlier historical time, but that is of no importance. The allegory is the key to the therapy. Lela made a breakthrough that day and was finally able to gain total control of her pain. Returning to health, she divorced her husband and later found work as a counselor in a pain clinic.

Continuing the Advancement of Medical Intuition

While at a meeting in April 1984, I met Caroline Myss, who introduced herself as one of those who could "read" human illness. A couple of months later, I phoned her and suggested that we test her accuracy. It turned out that she was correct 93 percent of the time in making psychological, physical, and biochemical diagnoses . . . as long as she didn't diagnose more than eight cases per day. It was a thrill to meet someone so accurate.

By 1988, Caroline and I were writing two books together: *AIDS: Passageway to Transformation* and *The Creation of Health.* We also began to do workshops together in the U.S., England, Scotland, and the Netherlands, and she has since gone on to become a best-selling author herself.

From the beginning of our work together, Caroline's belief that we have a purpose in life—a purpose to use the power within us responsibly, wisely, and lovingly—significantly resonated with me. It was the very essence of conscientiousness, something we both deeply believe in.

It was a joy to mentor her and contribute to her training. We spent countless hours discussing cases, clarifying medical terminology, traveling and presenting together, and in general talking a lot about how we could advance and help this profession. Toward this end, in the late 1990s Caroline and I established a comprehensive training course for individuals who were interested in becoming medical intuitives.

We went on to establish the American Board of Scientific Medical Intuition (ABSMI) to provide training in this field, leading to a board certification for those who were capable of passing the exam. As cofounders, Caroline and I wanted to ensure that standards were being met, but it turned out that few people were willing to put in the dedicated time for study and preparation that it took to be able to pass the final exam.

However, throughout the process, many of the students we worked with as part of the ABSMI program did become quite proficient as counseling intuitives, and many have gone on to use their gifts in that way. To be considered a fully competent medical intuitive, you must be able to make accurate physical, mental, or emotional diagnoses of recognized medical disorders, diseases, or illnesses.

Could Crystals Be Used for Healing?

Another field of study that I took great interest in was the power of crystals. In late 1987, I was approached by Lynn "Buck" Charlson, who asked if I would study the effects of crystals on healing. Buck Charlson was a brilliant man, a prolific inventor and innovator within the field of hydraulics, and he was also the founder of The Life Science Foundation. He said that if I agreed to study crystals, he would give me a research grant.

I spent months pondering the issue. On one occasion, I had a very strong psychic intuition that placing crushed sapphire crystal over the heart would eliminate the need for bypass surgery. As tempting as that concept was, I am a neurosurgeon, not a cardiologist or cardiac surgeon. And since cardiac surgery is one of the sacred money cows in medicine, and I was not a specialist in that field, I felt it best to ignore the suggestion! Instead, I opted to do research on the possibility of imprinting crystals to enhance happiness.

The following is a summary of that first successful project, which was one of the first of 12 research grants from the

Charlson Foundation and later through The Life Science Foundation. Throughout those years, I visited Buck outside Minneapolis about four times each year to discuss our research endeavors and findings.

Eventually, I did settle on using a stone for healing energy, but not sapphire. Instead, I chose quartz crystal, which is piezoelectric. This means that when you put pressure on quartz, it creates electricity, indicating to me that it could also receive, store, and transmit electromagnetic energy, which suited my needs for this study. The human body is similar to this mineral, because it's largely piezoelectric, especially in bones, muscles, tendons, and intestines.

I already knew that we could help 85 percent of depressed patients come out of depression through our two-week therapeutic program using education, music, exercise, autogenic training, transcranial electrical stimulation, and photostimulation (lights). Now I wondered, *What results could we get using crystals?*

For Buck's study, I enrolled 200 patients with depression. Throughout the two weeks, I worked with each patient in groups of 12 to 15 in order to develop a personal-healing phrase for each of them. Each phrase needed to include healing qualities with six or fewer words and an image of healing. Subsequent groups followed the same procedure. On the last day of each two-week session, patients were given a shaped quartz crystal or a placebo glass crystal. In this double-blind study, the nurse who distributed the crystals and glass did not know who received which one.

Once patients had the glass or quartz crystal in their hands, I instructed them on how to imprint it. They were to pass it through a candle flame with the intent of erasing any information in the crystal. Then with each of three deep breaths, they blew into their crystal while mentally repeating to themselves their specific healing phrase and visualizing their image. Then each patient placed the crystal (or placebo) into a small, white-satin pouch and wore it around the neck during the day. For the first week, they were asked to re-imprint it daily by following the same routine, and then to imprint it once a week thereafter.

After three months, the patients came back for a follow-up evaluation. Of the 200 patients, 85 percent believed they received the real quartz crystal, even though they knew they had only a 50 percent chance. Nonetheless, the results were remarkable. Only 18 percent (about average for a placebo) of those who received glass crystals were still out of depression, but *70 percent* of those who received the real quartz crystal were still out of depression. This study proved—beyond any reasonable doubt—that quartz could assist in healing. In fact, I don't know of any antidepressant drug that comes even close to that effectiveness!

The World Beyond What We Can See

There are many more alternative therapies that I have explored and used for myself and my patients over the years. I have written whole books and compendiums on many of them, including *Energy Medicine, Medical Intuition, Sacred Healing,* and *Life Beyond 100,* but it's not my intent to give an exhaustive discussion here on all of them.

Suffice it to say that alternative therapists, medical intuitives, and psychics in general get their inspiration in many different ways. For me, I would very often get an inkling of what was wrong or what was going on with a patient far beyond what I could have known given my training—or by reading their lab results or referring to what they told me. Other times, I would get more than just a hunch of an idea; rather, I would have actual conversations back and forth with angelic guides who identified themselves to me, sometimes by a name, sometimes just as my teacher.

Often I heard just a few sentences, but at times these conversations going on in my head would continue for up to an hour. These bursts of inspiration frequently come to me when I'm meditating, but not always. Sometimes, ideas just download into my head while I am feeding the animals on the farm or sitting in a meeting—anywhere at any time.

Virtually all of my own innovations—the 12 patents I have to my name that are related to pain therapy and the new products and supplements that I have developed—came about first from a point of divine inspiration. I would then use my scientific training to devise research studies that would prove and further develop what I had been intuitively given. Or in the case of my patients, my instincts would be validated in the course of my treatment of that individual.

Like so many of my colleagues in the holistic-medicine field, I have been blessed with being able to tap into the wisdom of the ages because I am open to it. But I firmly believe (as did Edgar Cayce and so many other leading thinkers) that all people in the world have intuition available to them as a tool to use in their lives. Some of us have just developed this skill to a higher degree than others.

I have been given and tested so many concepts throughout my career and done so much research that it has filled 29 books, and I'm sure that I have enough for 29 more. But most important to our discussions in this particular book are the practical life-style changes that we all can make that will lead us to a longer, healthier, and more conscientious life, and that is where we are going next.

ᴗᴗᴗ ᴗᴗᴗ

CHAPTER SIX

LIFESTYLE CHANGES THAT INCREASE HEALTH AND HAPPINESS

Using Your Conscientiousness to Avoid an Early Grave

So what is it that you *don't* understand about dying? I've often wondered about this, because so many people today just seem to be barreling full-steam ahead toward an early grave, completely oblivious! Perhaps they think that it won't happen to them, but you know what—none of us are getting out alive!

If death will happen, and it's not usually all that pleasant, why not try to avoid it as long as possible? Why not try to keep yourself in the best possible shape right up to the end, and then when it's time to go, you can wave good-bye with no regrets, suffering no pain, and on your own terms? That's my plan!

You can do this, too. It just takes some understanding of what's involved and that thing called *conscientiousness* I've been talking about. I believe that you can avoid a premature death—and stay healthy in mind and body right up until the end—just by taking a few conscientious steps each day.

But before getting to the best practices for our body, mind, and spirit, let me take a few steps back and give some context here. How did the human race get to this dismal state of health anyway? I believe that our current society, the medical industry itself, and industrialization have been conspiring against us. Once we understand more about this bigger picture—what has really happened to us as humans—I think we'll find that making a few lifestyle adjustments now is well worth the payoff that we'll enjoy later in life.

The State of the Union Has Been Falling Apart

So how did we in the U.S. arrive at the current state of physical, emotional, and spiritual dysfunction? I have a strong suspicion that the majority of Americans were motivated and working at a reasonable pace to achieve the American dream until the end of World War II. But over the subsequent two decades, the seeds of failure increased steadily.

As an example, prior to WWII, 95 percent of the food grown for consumption came from within 50 miles of where it was consumed. People ate real food—fresh fruits, vegetables, and meats grown locally—as their primary diet, they didn't even know what junk food was. Even lower-income individuals had adequate food.

But then came one of the first human-made plagues when pesticides such as DDT (dichlorodiphenyltrichloroethane) were introduced during the 1940s. Also around this time, nuclear energy arrived on the scene—one of the most serious threats to the survival of humanity that had ever been experienced. From those two elements, many more dominos began to fall, more or less in the following order.

Water was no longer sacred. First chlorine was introduced, which was bad enough, but then fluoride was added to drinking water, forever poisoning the body and mind. Pesticides, herbicides, and chemical poisons grew in numbers and reach, contaminating our agricultural land and running off into our waterways.

Then we had to face contamination from nuclear testing, bombing, and nuclear plants. Few of us could conceive of what havoc this technology would bring upon the world.

But at that point, government regulations of life itself were everywhere, and on the home front we were also experiencing the gradual industrialization of food and the death of the family farm. Coupled with that, we then saw the rise of fast-food restaurants and other junk foods influencing the population to replace real food with virtual food—products made with artificial ingredients that were never intended to nourish the human body.

Then enter the proliferation of television in general, and we became a nation glued to our screens as we sat on our backsides. We gave up reading for pleasure and walking to the store, and we also seemed to give up self-responsibility for our own health and well-being, because the government seemed so willing to do it for us! If only we knew then how they were going to screw it up. More people might have spoken up and organized a protest in the streets.

But by this time, physical activity and exercise had fallen out of any kind of favor, and the poor diets we were eating were causing us to pack on the pounds until the obesity crisis reared its head in the 1990s—which we're still struggling with 20 years later. Perhaps we didn't hear the wake-up call because we were glued to the tube or our computer screens.

Did anybody think to look up and see the government, insurance industry, and PharmacoMafia (my term for the pharmaceutical industry) taking complete control of medicine? I did. I saw the hijack happening, and so did many individuals in the medical field and holistic movement, but there wasn't much we could do about it. We tried to call them on it, but we did not control the money, and therefore did not control the power.

Imagine my shock and disbelief as a doctor when pharmaceuticals began advertising in print, on TV, and eventually all over the Internet, convincing most people that serious complications from their medications are merely side effects! I hate to be the bearer of bad news, my dear readers, but *death is not a side effect!* Imagine the audacity of drug manufacturers saying, at the end of so many of their long, rambling lists of side effects on their warning labels, "May cause death."

In the midst of society moving forward at warp speed, we also began to feel the fallout of the destruction of the nuclear family, as divorce rates rose and the number of teen and single-parent pregnancies increased. More and more of us became dependent on government handouts, and this started a cycle of poverty that seems to grip families like a vice for generations.

These are just some of the many manifestations of the widespread loss of conscientiousness with which we as individuals and as a society are now struggling. We have lost our way and our willpower at personal, internal, and transcendent levels.

But Don't Give Up! There Is Good News!

Before you begin to get depressed from the gloom and doom that I just listed, let's consider that by taking a conscientious approach to your own life and health, you can turn around this chaos.

Research tells us that if Americans were nonsmokers, carried normal weight, did some exercise each day, and followed good nutritional guidelines, their life span would increase at least 18 to 20 years! Likewise, it's clear from the research that inactivity, poor nutrition, obesity, and smoking often lead to damaged health for years *before* death.

Right now, the average life expectancy for Americans is 74.5 years for men and 80.5 for women. Man or woman, you lose six years at the end if you're a smoker and another six if you're obese or inactive.

Surely you would not want to die young or have the last ten years of your life full of illness and suffering if you could help it, right? The bottom line is that your health today and tomorrow is in your control; it is the result of habits, behavior, beliefs, attitudes, and your ancestors!

Personally, I have conscientiously chosen healthy habits, and I expect to remain healthy for many more years. I challenge you to choose wisely and enjoy all your remaining time on this planet. Here's the critical information that will help you achieve that:

10 Smart Steps to Keep You Alive (and Well!)

I have advised more than 30,000 patients over the years to follow these steps. In doing so, they were able to overcome pain and depression, and 85 percent of them got back on a solid path to wellness. You can increase your longevity by conscientiously taking the following steps yourself. More details follow, but here is the basic checklist for a long and healthy life!

1. Keep your body mass index (BMI) between 18 and 24.

2. Eat at least five (but preferably seven) servings of real fruits and vegetables daily.

3. Exercise a minimum of 30 minutes, 5 days a week (an hour is even better).

4. Do not smoke.

5. Get an adequate amount of sleep each night.

6. Practice at least 20 minutes each day of self-regulation, such as with the autogenic training method explained in the previous chapter.

7. Keep a positive attitude toward yourself, your life, and others.

8. Develop a strong social network of friends and loved ones.

9. Enjoy sex with a loving partner or by yourself; it releases tension and raises oxytocin.

10. When your diet can't supply everything you need, take some basic nutritional supplements that have been made under high-quality standards.

A Conscientious Diet Is a Good Diet

Let's face it: The number one preventable cause of premature death is obesity! A poor diet and inactivity are what most often create weight problems and disease. Only one-third of Americans today have a healthy body weight, one-third are overweight, and another third are just plain fat—obese! As I just mentioned, a healthy body weight is a BMI of 18 to 24, and this range allows for the wide variety of skeletal and muscular differences.

Note that whatever your height, 40 pounds or more of extra weight puts you immediately in the obese category, where the risks to your health and longevity are tremendously magnified.

In its simplest form, good nutrition is eating a wide variety of real food. Forty-five percent of all food consumed in the United States is fast food, which is all junk that's loaded with monosodium glutamate and other toxins. I went to McDonald's back in the 1960s, took one bite, and spit it out. I do not trust anything from any fast-food restaurant.

In grocery stores, 60 percent of all items are junk because they are made out of artificial ingredients. If it comes in a package and has more than one basic, easily recognizable ingredient and salt, it probably is not real food! As much as I prefer organic options, I do not trust all of those either. Know where it was grown and packaged—that is your best bet.

Many people also forget that proteins are the most essential of all foods. You cannot make DNA without them. You can make carbohydrates and fats from them, and, of course, most protein foods contain some fat. In order of quality, I consider the following high-quality proteins very healthy for you and to be enjoyed in variety and moderation each day: eggs, fish, cheese (especially goat cheese), fowl, beef, venison, rabbit, buffalo, and pork. Incidentally, there are ten absolutely essential amino acids, which you must eat in order to be healthy.

Additionally, the widespread deficiency of taurine in 84 percent of my patients suggests that many people are not eating adequate animal protein. Taurine is not in any vegetable food, but it is essential to maintaining the normal electrical charge on cell walls; it works synergistically with magnesium to maintain electrical balance.

As for meal planning in the ideal diet, I recommend that adults eat the following each day: one super salad; two other vegetables; two fruits; one or two servings of the good starches (not essential, but okay to eat); one serving of the highest-quality animal proteins (at least three or four times each week, which is essential for getting an adequate amount of vitamin B_{12}); and up to one serving of the four other good protein foods that I just mentioned, such as eggs, cheese, and beans, especially on days when you don't eat the higher-quality ones. If you do not eat one of the meats listed or eggs, then you should add yeast on those days for balance. But in terms of flavor, I have not tasted any yeast that compares well with any of the real animal foods! And, yes, yeast is just as much a living organism as any animal!

Please remember that added fats are also important for the body. I recommend that you include up to two tablespoons of fat in your daily diet, especially with meals that don't have a starch. My preferred fat choices are butter, olive oil, or coconut oil.

Condiments and herbs not only taste amazing but are very good for the body. There are scores of these marvelous tasty treats, most of which are loaded with antioxidants and great minerals. My favorites are cinnamon, turmeric, coriander, cumin, ginger, rosemary, thyme, mint, pimentón (a smoked Spanish paprika), and oregano. The other great seasoning agents are onions and garlic, which may be eaten as a serving of vegetables or used as seasonings, and are very versatile and good for you. You can also eat various seaweed products, if you like them.

With this as a guide for nutrition, there is no need for desserts. However, if you aren't overweight and are otherwise healthy, then a dessert once a week is fine. Personally, I enjoy one ounce of dark chocolate (70 percent or more of cocoa) as a treat after dinner about four times a week or so. Dark chocolate has been proven to be good for your health and is without the ill effects or high sugar content that's present in other kinds of chocolate products.

Five Tests Well Worth Taking

Under the model of becoming a conscientious citizen, you now are coming to realize that you are responsible for taking care of your own health. I agree that you should use your common sense to consult with a medical professional when you feel that you have something very serious to deal with, but most of the time it's just as helpful to apply your own initiative and seek natural methods of prevention and treatment for most ailments and conditions.

Part of the due diligence of taking good care of yourself, in addition to eating well and exercising, are five important tests that are known to detect problems. The issues highlighted by these tests are ones that can be easily corrected before they cause illness.

— I feel that perhaps the most critical test is for high-sensitivity C-reactive protein (hs-CRP). This test measures inflammation in the body and can detect things that range from a low-grade gum infection to serious issues like gallbladder or pelvic infections. The normal range is between one and three, but optimal is below one. (Anger can also cause elevated levels.) If your hs-CRP is at a one or above, you'll need to do a comprehensive physical exam. Taking antioxidants such as astaxanthin at 12 mg daily, which is my favorite, is one of the best ways to lower hs-CRP. And, as you will learn when we discuss the Ring of Crystal, stimulating that circuit can lower free radicals and inflammation better than any other approach I know.

— The second test I suggest is the homocysteine blood test. Homocysteine is an abnormal protein that, when elevated above 7.5 mg/L, leaves a person susceptible to heart attack, stroke, cancer, and Alzheimer's disease. It is easily corrected with specific supplements, in this case extra B_{12} and folic acid. Remember, any homocysteine level above 7.5 mg/L is risky!

— The third recommended test is for free radicals in your urine. This one measures the extent of cell death that is caused by excessive chemical oxidation, which again is easily fixed. For this, I would recommend Crystal Bliss essential oil blend, which is explained further in Chapter Seven. Although high intakes of antioxidants may reduce free radicals, I have found levels of two or above on the Oxidata test for malondialdehyde in 99 percent out of hundreds of individuals. The single best way to reduce free radicals is daily stimulation of the Ring of Crystal. Malondialdeyde is actually the metabolic breakdown of the fat layer that is around cells—in other words, it represents the cells killed by free radicals!

— As part of your health regime, the fourth test that I recommend is to check your levels of DHEA, which, as you'll recall, is the most essential hormone in the body. It's usually too low or deficient in the majority of people over the age of 40, but there are four safe, natural approaches to restoring DHEA, which we reviewed in Chapter Two. Be sure to check free DHEA, not DHEA sulfate! Incidentally, the only accurate lab is Quest Diagnostic Nichols Institute in Capistrano, California!

— The fifth test you should consider taking is one that measures your cholesterol level. Cholesterol is the foundation for most hormones and the nervous system. Your body needs and manufactures cholesterol constantly, but high levels are not good for you. Just ten minutes of stress produces more cholesterol than you get from eating two eggs!

Speaking of eggs, while there are studies of many kinds about them, I believe there is no credible evidence that they are harmful to you, unless you are specifically allergic to egg protein. The cholesterol contained in them is perfectly balanced by lecithin. The most remarkable report is of a man who ate 25 eggs daily and had a cholesterol reading of 125—which is quite good! Obviously, eggs—and their yolks—didn't cause him cholesterol problems, and they shouldn't affect you negatively either.

Myths and Truths about Cholesterol and Fats

Where in the world can you eat food high in fat and get away with it? In just about every country of the world apparently, and there is lots of research to prove it. Medicine's greatest error in the past 50 years has been the war on cholesterol. This may seem surprising, but many studies show that people who eat more cholesterol and saturated fat than their peers also weigh less than those same individuals.

This is because increased weight gain and elevated cholesterol levels are invariably correlated. Furthermore, those who eat the least amount of saturated fat and cholesterol seem to have twice the death rate compared to their peers with diets higher in these elements.

In Okinawa, Japan, where inhabitants eat large amounts of pork and cook with lard, the average life expectancy of women is 84. It is interesting, too, that Jews who live in Yemen, who intake fat solely of animal origin but eat no sugar, have minimal rates of heart disease and diabetes. Yemenite Jews who have been transplanted to Israel tend to eat more margarine, vegetable oils, and sugar than their traditional cousins at home in Yemen, and with that change in diet come resultant higher levels of heart disease and diabetes in those living in Israel.

Residents of northern India eat 17 times more animal fat than those in southern India, yet the southern Indians have a seven times greater incidence of heart disease. And while the African Masai eat mostly milk and beef blood, heart disease is rare and cholesterol is low among them.

Residents of Crete obtain 70 percent of their calories from lamb, sausage, and goat cheese and have very low rates of heart disease. The Inuit people (also sometimes called Eskimos) are relatively free of heart disease, despite a high intake of fat, as long as they avoid sugar.

The Chinese, who consume great quantities of nonhomogenized milk, have half the rate of heart disease as those who eat little animal fat. In the country of Georgia, those who eat the fattiest kinds of meats actually live the longest.

The incidence of death from coronary artery disease in France is 55 percent lower than in the U.S. despite its citizens' high intake of butter, eggs, cream, and liver pâté. Indeed, in the areas of that country with the highest consumption of goose and duck liver, the incidence of coronary heart disease is a striking 76 percent below that of Americans.

The Relationship Between Carbs and Cholesterol

When you look at research done around the world, you see that this really comes down to a truth that few in North America seem willing to accept—namely, it is carbohydrates that make you fat, not eating fat! Beef fat is considerably better at improving cholesterol than equal calories from bread, potatoes, and pasta. And nonhydrogenated pork lard is even better than other shortenings.

As you seek to understand all this, here is how carbohydrates affect the body. The problem with them is in how they are related to the glycemic index (GI). Sugar has a GI of 100, and all other foods are measured against this. White bread is 97, which is almost as high as sugar itself, while nuts have a GI of only 15. This means that nuts raise blood sugar at only 15 percent the rate of sugar.

Eating foods with a high GI leads to insulin release, which increases fat storage in your body. High dairy fat decreases insulin resistance. So that Super Big Gulp soda that seems so appealing on your drive home from work is just 64 ounces of pure junk, containing 48 teaspoons of sugar with 292 calories for fat production. Artificial sweeteners, such as aspartame, are even worse; studies show that aspartame actually prevents weight loss and increases appetite, which most people don't understand at all. Don't be fooled.

It is also a fact that trans fats—hydrogenated margarine, shortening, and most peanut butters, to name a few—are at least as serious of a threat to causing high cholesterol as anything else. These ingredients are found in many pastries, doughnuts, deep-fried foods, crackers, and fast food. They increase insulin release and are associated with heart disease, cancer, immune dysfunction, sterility, growth problems, osteoporosis, and hearing loss. Not all peanut butter is bad for you, though. As part of my own conscientious nutrition regime, I take a tablespoon or two of natural peanut butter in my diet with no ill effects.

Here is one of the biggest cautions I can offer. I personally would not turn to drugs in order to control or reduce cholesterol problems. While statin drugs, which are the PharmacoMafia's current answer to cholesterol problems, can modestly reduce cholesterol, they clobber the liver and immune function.

Instead, here are some natural ways to bring down your cholesterol and control your overall weight. Start with any kind of physical exercise, and build up to one hour daily. Ensure a high intake of nonstarchy vegetables and fruits daily, striving for seven servings. Enjoy a program of deep-relaxation exercises (self-regulation) for 20 minutes daily.

Also, avoid hydrogenated fats of all kinds, and don't drink soda or eat at fast-food restaurants. Stay away from homogenized milk, and instead drink at least two quarts of nonchlorinated water each day. I recommend using only butter and olive, coconut, sesame, and flaxseed oils as added fats in your diet.

If your cholesterol is still above 200 after six weeks on the above regimen, consider adding one of the following supplements to your diet: timed-release niacin, 500 mg at each meal; beta-sitosterol, 400 mg at each meal; arginine, 5 grams daily with 2.5 grams citrulline in timed-release capsules; taurine, 3 to 4 grams daily; or lecithin granules, four heaping tablespoons daily.

Exercise: The Key to Health and Happiness

I have been an exercise buff all my life. As a child, I did the Charles Atlas dynamic isometric exercise program, and I was lifting weights even before medical school. Today, I still do 75 to 90 minutes of exercise daily, but no weight lifting. Three years ago, at the age of 77, I did a treadmill stress test. It showed that my body was equal to most healthy 26-year-olds, so I live by my own advice, and it's a great life!

I tell you this not to boast, but to emphasize my belief that physical exercise is the single greatest boost to health and longevity. Time and time again, I have seen that when patients would start and stick with a good exercise program, they would overcome depression, stress, anxiety, and pain—and live longer lives.

When you exercise, you will suffer far fewer illnesses or ailments throughout your life, and you can stay away from unnecessary pharmaceuticals, such as antidepressants. No drugs are free of side effects, and many cause worse situations than they were intended to cure. For example, a March 15, 2011, article published in *The American Journal of Psychiatry* reported that when researchers studied the cases of more than 24,000 patients who had suffered strokes, they found that the prior use of antidepressants was associated with a 48 percent increased stroke risk! This is just one example—and you could easily find hundreds more—but I don't want to dwell on the negatives.

Physical exercise has all kinds of positive aspects, but let me share just a few. I totally believe that it is the single best and safest treatment for mild to major depression, even in those people who are resistant to drug therapy, and it is also the best and safest treatment for anxiety. Getting your body moving every day also reduces stress, hostility, and anger.

There are all kinds of research studies that show how exercise improves cognitive thinking at all ages and helps prevent Alzheimer's disease and dementia. It reduces fibromyalgia symptoms more than any known drug, and, in fact, a good regimen reduces mortality at any age, especially from heart disease. In addition, you can improve immune function, keep from becoming overweight, and reduce your risk of diabetes. I could go on and on— the benefits are endless.

As for what you choose to do for your own program, to some extent, it does not matter what you do for exercise. In general, a brisk walk is superb. Aim to build up to a minimum of two miles in 30 minutes, which is not really that hard. Various yoga techniques and exercises are excellent as well. When you can't get out, I find that treadmills are good. My favorite one is a HealthRider, which works out every muscle in your body except your face. Walking or jogging in a swimming pool is another outstanding way to get your body moving.

If you are resistant to exercise, try bouncing—even while watching TV. Build up to three minutes of bouncing ten times a day. Your immune system, mood, and overall health will improve immensely just by getting yourself moving. You can bounce on a small trampoline or in place. Just do an Internet search for "Bounce with Dr. Shealy" on YouTube to see how easy it is.

Proper Sleep Is Necessary for Health

As more and more people are reporting sleep disorders, we are seeing all kinds of sleep clinics and drug-based solutions popping up everywhere. I would suggest that making personal lifestyle changes should be your first line of defense before seeing the doctor, unless you are very ill or worried about something more serious.

There is quite a bit of scientific evidence that sleep deficiencies are a major contributing factor to the obesity crisis. Over and over, studies are showing that too little sleep is linked to weight gain.

There are various theories as to why this is so, but there may be three primary reasons why getting proper sleep helps you manage your weight better. If you are going to bed at a decent hour each night, you have fewer evening hours to snack on poor food choices you might otherwise seek. Some other scientists say that too little sleep produces excess stress and causes havoc with hunger hormones and the body's ability to process sugars in food. Other experts claim that lack of proper sleep is a vicious circle—you are just too tired when waking up to feel like going to the gym or working out, thus your body packs on the pounds from inactivity! Whatever the reason, a conscientious person knows that it is best to go to bed and wake up at the same time each day, getting a minimum of seven good hours of sleep. As for getting to sleep, the wisdom of your mother is still valid: Why not try a glass of warm milk?

I also recommend listening to relaxing music, the gentle sounds of nature, or autogenic-training CDs in order to calm your mind, body, and spirit. I would not recommend drinking anything with caffeine after the noon hour if getting to sleep is an issue. And of course, one of the best ways to drift off to a blissful sleep is using Air Bliss essential oil blend applied to the Ring of Air points on the body before bed (Air Bliss is explained further in the next chapter).

Selecting Supplements That Work for You

When it comes to nutritional supplements, it depends very much on what your system still may need that it's not getting from your normal diet, what your body might need to help protect itself from illness, or what's necessary to recover from physical concerns that you may have developed.

But in general terms, the supplements I recommend most often happen to be these:

- B complex (25 mg daily) and some trace minerals—critical for brain and nerve function.

- Magnesium lotion (2 teaspoons twice daily on the skin)—this is essential to 350 different enzymes in the body, and it's absorbed far more effectively through the skin than by swallowing a capsule.

- Astaxanthin (10 mg daily)—this is the single best overall antioxidant.

- Vitamin D$_3$ (50,000 units once a week)—the single best boost to immune function. Doing this will prevent at least 80 percent of viral infections!

- Omega-3 (1,000 to 2,000 mg daily)—this is essential for artery and brain function.

- Lithium orotate (15 to 20 mg daily)—essential for serotonin optimization, this stabilizes mood and helps deal with trauma.

The Path to a Long Life Really Starts with Love

Thank you for sticking with me through a chapter about life and death, which can both be pretty heavy topics. What it ultimately comes down to is that in order to enjoy optimal health throughout your life, and do good for yourself and others, you need love—and you also need to love others unconditionally.

When you truly love yourself, you will care enough to make the necessary changes you've just learned about. I could certainly write a full book on the healing power of love (and I probably will one day), but for now I'd just like you to accept this premise and move with me to the next chapter, where we will discuss ways to stay positive and blissful all your days on this Earth. I invite you to let that bliss give you the chance to open your heart and truly love yourself, just in case you are not completely there yet.

✧ ✧ ✧ ✧ ✧ ✧

CHAPTER SEVEN

BOOSTING OXYTOCIN AND DHEA THROUGH BLISS THERAPIES

As you have been reading along, you have heard me mention the Sacred Rings and the Bliss therapies a few times. I have to say that these have been among the most effective and exciting innovative therapies that I have ever developed. This series of treatments is based on the wisdom of the ages, since I got the inspiration for them through a progression of divine messages over a period of the past 10 to 12 years.

This chapter introduces how I developed these therapies, how to use them, and what each one is best suited to achieve. In combination with a conscientious lifestyle, I have seen firsthand how these therapies can extend our lives, with the focus on maximizing the number of healthy years we enjoy.

In particular, the Ring of Air circuit (which I explain in this chapter) has shown incredible power to change people's lives. For a huge majority of the unhappy, unfulfilled individuals who are suffering from a wide variety of emotional disorders, Air Bliss appears to help at least 90 percent of people overcome depression and manage themselves better just by activating the body points that correspond to the Ring of Air.

In addition to trials and research studies that I conduct with regard to all my products and therapies, I regularly receive lots of interesting feedback in the form of e-mails, letters, and testimonials.

One woman recently wrote to me that her 60-year-old son who had been miserably angry and depressed all his life is now happy and at peace after beginning the practice of applying Air Bliss essential oils each morning and evening!

As I often say, nothing works in 100 percent of people. We cannot even be sure that someone is alive or dead without taking it to the Supreme Court! But as this book has been clearly demonstrating, conscientiousness begins with reasonable happiness, and Air Bliss is able to provide that foundation for those in need of it. This is one of the best first steps to becoming the dependable, productive, and creative individual you want to be and allowing you to have the energy and passion to do good for others.

Medical Intuition at Work Once Again

I believe that the inspiration for the advances made possible through the Five Sacred Rings came to me because I was in a unique frame of mind and in a position to test and refine them through my research and wide network of connections. These therapies are a natural extension of my medical training and my experience in energy work, holistic medicine, and aroma acupuncture. I must say that my skills in this life were ideally matched to put these therapies into motion.

Here's the path I have been on. Over the past dozen years or so, I intuitively became aware of five human circuits, which I was told were to be called the Sacred Rings. Each one consists of a number of specific points in the human body that, when activated in sequence, provide relief from a wide range of human conditions and ailments.

From the point of inspiration, I worked with my inner guide to glean more and more details in order to understand fully and perfect each therapy. As I meditated and asked for further direction, I would be told by my guide the purpose of the ring that was being given.

My job was to define the exact acupuncture points and, except for the first one, to use my own intuition to determine the biochemical effect each ring would be able to influence. The first one, the Ring of Fire, was unique in that I knew what I wanted to influence. As the other Rings were given to me, my guide never indicated what the biochemical effect would be. I will discuss this further a bit later.

Enhancing DHEA with the Ring of Fire

The timing for this particular intuitive inspiration came just as I had begun researching DHEA. As you will recall from our previous chapters, virtually all the depressed patients that I have seen in my clinical days have had either low or deficient levels of DHEA.

As described earlier, almost all people gradually develop low or deficient levels of this important hormone, from a high point of DHEA at about age 25, and then gradually decreasing with age. By age 80, most people have less than 10 percent of what they had at age 30; and since DHEA deficiency is found in every known illness, there is a benefit in finding ways to keep this depletion from happening or rejuvenating it in individuals who are severely lacking it.

Taking DHEA is not an optimal way to replenish it, as it may stimulate activity in dormant cancer cells located in the breast, prostate, uterus, or ovaries. In general, if you have any condition that might be made worse by exposure to estrogen, it is not advisable to take this hormone. This is particularly true for estrogen-sensitive breast cancer, but DHEA is also not recommended for women suffering with uterine cancer, ovarian cancer, endometriosis, or uterine fibroids—or for men with prostate problems.

I had a feeling that natural progesterone should increase DHEA, so I tested it. Indeed, it did increase DHEA, but only at an average of 60 percent. While it sounds like a great advance, I soon realized that this method just did not do enough by itself to make a difference. Research showed that most people who are over 40 years of age have levels that are already 50 percent lower than the ideal DHEA levels. Normal levels should be in the range of 750 to 1,200 ng/dl in men and 500 to 980 ng/dl in women.

I reasoned that if these average patients would be starting at such depleted levels as 200, then even a 100 percent increase does not get us anywhere near the ideal levels that humans require.

It was at this point that the inspiration from my guide showed me the way. I was told that if I stimulated the points that connect the kidneys, gonads, adrenals, thyroid, and pituitary gland through a window of the sky point (there are 22 window of the sky points in acupuncture—these connect body and mind with the soul), then I could significantly raise the levels of human DHEA.

My challenge, then, was that since there is no point in Chinese cosmology that corresponds to the pituitary gland, I had to intuit it in order that this ring would become complete. Thus, the following series of points came to me, which I was told to call the Ring of Fire, and it has since proven effective in raising human DHEA levels, as well as helping migraines, rheumatoid arthritis, diabetic neuropathy, and depression—all disorders that are related to the fire element.

The Ring of Fire—Circuit Points in the Body

- **Kidney 3** (Stimulate or apply Fire Bliss oil behind the ankle bones, on the inside where the ankles touch when standing.)

- **Conception Vessel 2** (Stimulate or apply Fire Bliss oil on the center of the pubic bone.)

- **Conception Vessel 6** (Stimulate or apply Fire Bliss oil about a half inch below the umbilicus, which is the belly button.)

- **Conception Vessel 18** (Stimulate or apply Fire Bliss oil about two inches down from the top of the breast bone.)

- **Bladder 22** (Stimulate or apply Fire Bliss oil directly behind the belly button on your lower back, one inch to either side of the spine.)

- **Master of Heart 6** (Stimulate or apply Fire Bliss oil on the inside of the wrists about one inch up from the palms.)

- **Large Intestine 18** (Stimulate or apply Fire Bliss oil on the sides of the neck about one inch down from the mastoid bones, which lie just below the ears.)

- **Governing Vessel 20** (Stimulate or apply Fire Bliss oil to the point that's on the top and center of the skull, up from the ears.)

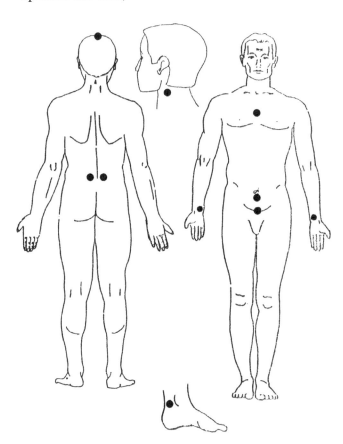

Results with Use of the Ring of Fire

Over a 12-week period, I found that stimulation of these points with 75 decibels of human DNA frequency (54 to 78 GHz), 3 minutes per pair of points daily, led to an average increase in DHEA of 60 percent (with a range between 30 and 100). This stimulation was done using the Shealy PainPro, which I talked about earlier. Incidentally, these patient results were *in addition to* what we achieved with the progesterone cream.

Later I discovered that a combination of vitamin C, methylsulfonylmethane (MSM), molybdenum, and beta-1,3-glucan raised DHEA another 60 percent. For ease, I put this combination together and began offering a formula called Dr. Shealy's Youth Formula, so patients could benefit from the right combination of these elements.

Furthermore, I also researched and tested the efficacy of magnesium chloride when applied transdermally (rubbed onto the skin). Sure enough, this also raised DHEA levels another 60 percent in the patients who tried it for this purpose.

Therefore, when these four techniques were applied together, DHEA was raised 250 percent over baseline, which was then enough to make a significant difference in the health of patients who were afflicted with obvious "fire" diseases.

These were some of the results we found when patients followed this regime:

- 70 percent of patients with rheumatoid arthritis, who had failed conventional medicine, improved dramatically.

- 75 percent of patients with frequent migraines showed a 75 percent reduction of frequency and severity of their headaches.

- 70 percent of depressed patients came out of depression.

- 70 percent of patients with chronic back pain improved.

- 80 percent of patients with diabetic neuropathy improved markedly from their pain, and at least 25 percent had improvement in sensory loss and were able to reduce their diabetic medications.

Activating the Ring of Fire with Essential Oil

While the therapeutic benefits of electrical stimulation were proven, I still found that patients did not wish to spend the 18 minutes daily that this therapy required. Feedback from test subjects was that this was just too much effort for most people.

With that in mind, I have since created Fire Bliss, which is a mixture of essential oils specifically for activating the healing properties of fire energy in the human body. Use of this essential oil blend has the potential to help thousands of individuals who suffer with rheumatoid arthritis, migraines, diabetic neuropathy, depression, and back pain. It is easily applied to the same circuit points listed above, but takes only about 30 seconds. I now call this approach *transcutaneous acupuncture*.

Another way to activate the Ring of Fire circuit is through listening to one of my CD recordings, which trains you to use your mind to trigger the healing power of this ring. It is basically an exercise for energizing the electrical battery of the body, since the Ring of Fire integrates the adrenals, chakras, and endocrine system.

Alternatively, you might consider a vigorous massage of these circuit points or tapping them to release their power. These methods take practice, but they can be quite effective for some people. Please note that each of these activation methods is possible for any of the five rings I have researched so far.

Inspiration for the Ring of Air

A few months after receiving inspiration about the Ring of Fire, my guide shared with me the Ring of Air, with the indication that this would stimulate "simultaneity of thought" (that is to say, it would raise one's intuition) and advance consciousness for mental creativity, symbolic thought, and mystical insight. Clinically, I was told that it would help hearing and tinnitus, and it would also calm anger and heal rage. The guide also said that this ring would be useful for autism and Down syndrome when it's used with the Ring of Earth, which he indicated would come to me much later.

As it turned out, I found that the initial details that came to me were just the tip of the iceberg for the incredible transformational change that the Ring of Air could actually produce once we started using and testing it.

The Ring of Air—Circuit Points in the Body

- **Spleen 1 A, bilaterally** (Stimulate or apply Air Bliss oil at the tip of each of the big toenails on the side of the toe that faces the other foot when standing normally.)

- **Liver 3, bilaterally** (Stimulate or apply Air Bliss oil to the top of each foot, between the big toe and second toe, just up from the web of the toes.)

- **Stomach 36, bilaterally** (Stimulate or apply Air Bliss oil to the top outside of each shinbone, as high as you can go just below the knee.)

- **Governing Vessel 1** (Stimulate or apply Air Bliss oil to the point at the very bottom of the spine.)

- **Lung 1, bilaterally** (Stimulate or apply Air Bliss oil under the bottom of the collarbone, on the right and left, as far out as you can go.)

- **Gallbladder 20, bilaterally** (Stimulate or apply Air Bliss oil to both sides of the back of the skull, halfway across the bottom from the mastoid bone, which lies just below the ears.)

- **Governing Vessel 16** (Stimulate or apply Air Bliss oil to the very top of the spine, just below the skull.)

- **Governing Vessel 20** (Stimulate or apply Air Bliss oil to the point that is on the top and center of the skull, up from the ears.)

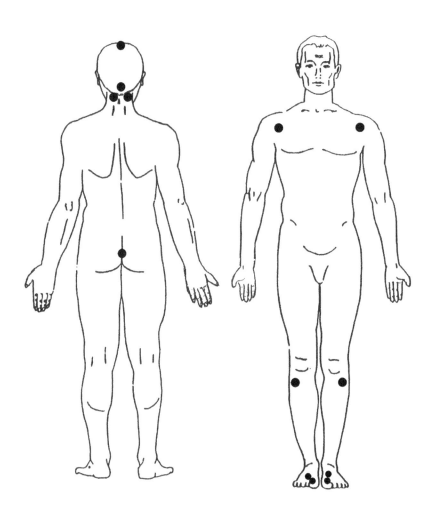

The Amazing Power of the Ring of Air

At first I wasn't sure what the Ring of Air would impact. But when I started working to develop this idea, I said to my research nurse, Vera, "We need to find out what the Ring of Air does."

So she asked me, "What do you want to measure?"

I blurted out, "Neurotensin. Call the lab and see whether they can measure neurotensin." At the time, I did not know anything about neurotensin. This is one of those situations where my intuition downloaded the word. We did the tests and found that its levels increased by up to 600 percent after the stimulation of the Ring of Air with GigaTENS (electrical stimulation at 54 to 78 billion cycles per second).

At that point, I researched further and learned that neurotensin markedly interrelates with growth hormones and insulin, as well as prolactin, which is a milk-releasing hormone. Neurotensin coordinates digestion (especially of fat), and it is both anti-nociceptive (pain relieving) and neuroleptic (anxiety reducing, tranquilizing).

Indeed, there are neuroleptic drugs that are major tranquilizers used to treat psychosis or induce anesthesia. The original tranquilizer, Thorazine, was the precursor for many more that came after. The first significant modern neuroleptic, ketamine, is an anesthetic and tranquilizer, and I'd done some original animal work on its effectiveness for pain physiology in 1965. This was yet another one of the many examples in my life where points of reference came up again in different ways!

Activating the Ring of Air with Essential Oil

Notwithstanding the extraordinary therapeutic benefits that were possible through electrical stimulation of the Ring of Air points, patients still preferred not to spend all of 21 minutes per day on this therapy. Considering that the test subjects were either depressed or in some kind of pain (or both) to start with, I felt that it was necessary to try to develop an easier, quicker solution.

Thus, I set out to create an Air Bliss mixture of essential oils that could activate the same level of healing and improvement that we saw through electrical stimulation. In just 30 seconds, Air Bliss starts to work, and it has turned out to be far more powerful than we even expected!

Placing Air Bliss oil on these specific body points significantly helps in relieving depression and anxiety, and early reports show improvement in autism, Asperger's syndrome, insomnia, and PTSD.

The Ring of Air's Ability to Raise Oxytocin

Some years after my work with the Ring of Air and neurotensin, I had a sudden realization that this ring could also raise oxytocin. I have now proven this to be true. As with so many good things in my life that have been brought to me by my wife, Chardy, I think that this particular realization had just as much to do with her as it did with my own inner guidance.

Looking back over my own life, I have been blessed in so many ways, including a wonderful marriage of more than 50 years and exceptionally good overall health. The two are indeed intrinsically interrelated, as I have described in earlier chapters.

Being married to such a highly conscientious person as Chardy meant that I had to be pretty darn organized for all those years. She would not let any of us slack off for very long on nutrition, exercise, or taking responsibility for ourselves, before gently (or sometimes not so gently) suggesting a correction back to basics.

Up until 2010, I fully expected that we would both live out our conscientious lives on our farm in Missouri, happily continuing to enjoy our children and grandchildren when they would come to visit and feeding our favorite horses every day. Given the success of our lives and careers, I felt that I could handle anything life might bring.

What I did not expect was Chardy's death. When she was suddenly given a very grave diagnosis, we pulled out every stop to try to restore her to health. I regret that she was unable to beat it, and I found that dealing with her loss was deeper and far more painful than I could have ever anticipated.

In the time since her passing, I have cried more than in the first 77 years of my life. I have used the Liss Cranial Stimulator more since her death than during the entire previous 25 years. It helps me immensely, as does Air Bliss, the essential oils mixture that I just described.

But here's the connection and next step. It was just a few weeks after Chardy's death, when I happened to find a few articles on oxytocin, the nurturing, bonding hormone. I instantly knew with such a strong intuition that seeing those articles had to be a download from my angelic guide, maybe even as a result of a nudge from Chardy.

Reading those articles, I came to realize that the Ring of Air must also raise oxytocin in the body, as well as neurotensin. I spent hours on the Internet, and finally found one paper reporting that oxytocin is released when neurotensin increases. I was so excited that I had difficulty sleeping that night.

Measuring and Proving the Connection to Oxytocin

It had been more than ten years since I first demonstrated that "Giga stimulation" (with the Shealy PainPro) of the Ring of Air strikingly raises neurotensin, but now I could see a natural link with oxytocin as well. Oxytocin is well known as the bonding or nurturing hormone, and I already knew that workshop participants almost universally reported feeling calm, relaxed, and detached after massaging, tapping, or applying Air Bliss to the Ring of Air points.

My research showed that oxytocin inadequacy has been reported in every known emotional and mental disorder, from autism, ADHD, addiction, depression, and OCD to schizophrenia. As was the case with neurotensin, it took me some time to find a lab for measuring oxytocin. Despite hundreds of papers on the general subject of, there seemed to be no commercial lab for testing human oxytocin levels. All the work had been done at universities, and I was finding the collection of data and measurement rather tedious.

Fortunately, I met Dr. Paul Durham through my friend Dr. Roger Cady. Roger's son Ryan worked at Dr. Durham's lab at Missouri State University. When I met with them, they agreed to do the lab tests for me at cost.

We began by measuring the oxytocin levels of ten volunteers, both before and after Giga stimulation of the Ring of Air circuit. Several days later, we measured oxytocin before and after the application of Air Bliss on the same points.

Giga stimulation of the Ring of Air raised oxytocin in eight of the participants—the same percent as our original findings with neurotensin! Air Bliss increased oxytocin in six of the participants.

Afterward, I evaluated the Air Bliss application in almost 100 individuals, and virtually all reported feeling calm, relaxed, and detached—free of anxiety. I expect this is a result of the combination of increased neurotensin and oxytocin.

It was then that I began a study of Air Bliss on the Ring of Air to test its effects on anxiety and depression, with a keen eye on raising conscientiousness, too. I reasoned that being calm, relaxed, and detached would allow a person to feel more at peace and able to focus on conscientiousness.

By this time, through everything I had seen and dealt with at the Shealy Pain Clinic for all those years, I sensed that the common root of all emotional problems was quite likely the result of oxytocin deficiency. This fit nicely with the findings that its treatments appear to help the gamut of emotional disturbances, including autism, ADHD, addiction, depression, OCD, and even schizophrenia. In one study I did there was a highly significant reduction in both anxiety and depression in 30 patients.

Patients' Stories Highlighting the Ring of Air

Many positive things come to pass through the use of the Ring of Air. One I remember fondly was Bruce, a very busy 3-year-old who accompanied his mother when she came to see me about her own health problems. Bruce was a typical child with ADHD, climbing up onto the windowsill, moving quickly and continuously.

I turned on the RelaxMate glasses, and he was instantly attracted to them, putting them on and enjoying the flashing lights. He remained quiet for the remainder of the time his mother was in my office, and I knew that I could help him in a number of ways. In fact, I have many notes from parents confirming the benefit of the RelaxMate glasses and the Ring of Air, which has helped them tremendously to calm down their children and control ADHD.

Another example was an 8-year-old boy with autism who was brought to me, able to speak only about 50 words. I showed his mother how to stimulate her son's body on the Ring of Air and Ring of Earth points, and within three weeks he was speaking 450 words. Within three months, he spoke fluently! Patients do not always experience such dramatic changes, but I have seen more than a few miraculous improvements in my many years in this field.

All ages can benefit from the Ring of Air therapy, which some people also use in combination with other products we offer. One particular war veteran has e-mailed me almost weekly about his experiences and those of his wife. Their example illustrates well how this kind of therapy can work for patients with serious challenges, so I asked him if I might quote him. This is the personal statement he sent back, which I very much enjoyed hearing:

> I've been using the Air Bliss now for close to four weeks. I'm using it every night and am sleeping better, as is my wife. As far as the PTSD nightmares, I've had only one, and it was mild. I find that my mood is improving, as is my ability to concentrate. My instincts are becoming

sharper again, which is a great help when doing community house calls to psychiatric clients.

He went on to describe how our products helped improve his life in a number of ways:

I usually meditate at night and use the Air Bliss and one of the other Sacred Rings. It's amazing how that combination improves my meditation, which helps in my writing. The PTSD is a condition that has caused my family and me some uncomfortable moments. My wife gives the Air Bliss tremendous credit for the improvement in me. I agree and just keep putting one foot in front of the other, one day at a time. Thank you for your kindness and friendship.

The Air Bliss is close to being empty, so I will be ordering the next bottle. My wife uses the Ring of Water and gets a tremendous benefit from it. We both use the Liss Cranial Stimulator every morning, and I personally like to use it in my office prior to the day's work. It really helps focus my mind.

The depression that can follow the PTSD nightmares is no longer an issue. It's my opinion that your devices can be of great help, and there are no side effects (but a calm relaxed feeling). I use the RelaxMate glasses normally at night and like them also. They tend to bring my mind to a focused, relaxed place, where positive thought comes easily, as does prayer and meditation.

This particular man found that, in conjunction with other therapeutic products, he was experiencing a new lease on life and renewed interest in getting back to work.

His summary of the experiences with these products has elements that I hear often, but not usually with such eloquence and clarity. He said in closing:

As your devices are holistic in nature, I wanted to be more thorough in my reporting of the results in using them. The nature of man is as a physical, mental, emotional, and spiritual being. The devices you have been guided to create have benefited me not only physically, mentally, and emotionally, but they are helping my wife. We speak often of the results we've had using these devices.

As of this writing, this man has continued to remain essentially free of PTSD for more than 18 months.

On any given day, I don't know what queries and responses I might get by phone, by e-mail, or via my radio show. I spend time during my workday consulting with other professionals, and I am always pleased to hear from them when they have hands-on feedback to share. Recently, I received the following note that speaks to the power of Air Bliss to raise oxytocin and allow people to form greater emotional connections and natural bonds.

In the words of one of these individuals: "I am a psychotherapist and passionate about energy psychology. I find my work deeply rewarding, being able to routinely facilitate dramatic, positive change for my clients. I got a similar result with Air Bliss to your medical colleague who thought he was already coping well with stress until he actually tried Air Bliss. The oxytocin enables me to be even more deeply empathic with my clients. Thanks for the great product."

Emotional Balancing with the Ring of Water

Moving on from the Ring of Air, the next ring I was given was the Ring of Water, which I was told by my guide was for emotional balance, edema, congestion, lowering cholesterol, and contacting the Christological heart—that is, the heart of the Christ consciousness.

When my guide mentioned the physical placements, I chose the appropriate acupuncture points. At that time, I also intuitively knew that it had to do with aldosterone, an adrenal hormone responsible for water and potassium balance.

Biochemically, the Ring of Water normalizes aldosterone when the body circuit is stimulated with GHz—that is to say, both high and low levels of aldosterone return to normal. The Ring of Water also helps with weight loss, but I figured out that it usually needs to be used in conjunction with the Ring of Fire in this case.

I now have shown that the Water Bliss essential oil blend also normalizes aldosterone. I can see already that it will be helpful in clinical situations where both high and low aldosterone levels are in need of being rebalanced.

When patients used GigaTENS on both the fire and water circuit points, they lost 8 to 11 pounds each week. But after a month or so, many of them discontinued the therapy because the process seemed to take too long (about 40 minutes each day). But of course, the essential oils take only a few minutes and work just as well.

Recently, a young woman used only Water Bliss, because she did not like the smell of Fire Bliss. She lost 25 pounds in four months and is continuing the daily routine, since it takes only 30 seconds to apply the oil. Another young man with tremendous swelling of his legs for many years has had amazing reduction in the swelling through the use of Water Bliss.

The Ring of Water—Circuit Points in the Body

- **Spleen 4** (Run your fingers back along the long bones of the big toe until you reach a joint on the inside of the foot. Wiggle your toes to know when you are on the joint, and then stimulate or apply Water Bliss oil.)

- **Conception Vessel 14** (Stimulate or apply Water Bliss oil on the center of your abdomen, just below the breastbone.)

- **Governing Vessel 8** (Stimulate or apply Water Bliss oil on your back at the point directly behind the previous point—Conception Vessel 14—so that you are putting it in the center over the spine.)

- **Bladder 13** (Lay your hands on the tops of your shoulders. The tips of your long fingers, placed to touch 1 inch to either side of the spine, will now be on Bladder 13; stimulate or apply Water Bliss oil.)

- **Heart 6** (Feel the space between two tendons on the outer wrists, just beyond the palm of the long bone of the small fingers; this is Heart 6—stimulate or apply Water Bliss oil here.)

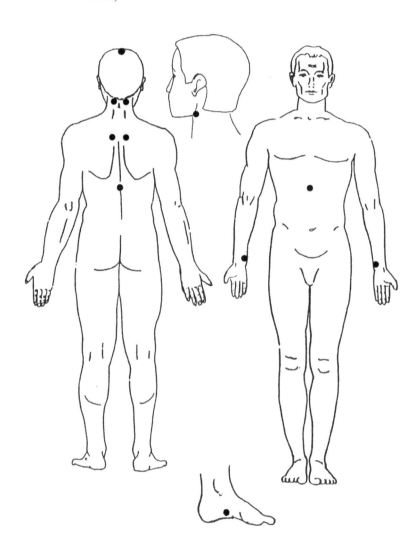

- **Bladder 10** (Put your middle fingers a half inch to both sides of the center of the spine, an inch below the skull; stimulate or apply Water Bliss oil.)

- **Triple Heater 16** (Turn your head to the left side and feel the back of the sternocleidomastoid muscle that becomes tight on the right side of your neck, and massage the back of that muscle just below the mandible (lower jaw); then turn your head to the right and do the same thing on the similar area in your left neck. Or apply Water Bliss oil to both points.)

- **Governing Vessel 20** (Stimulate or apply Water Bliss oil to the point that is on the top center of the skull, up from the ears.)

Pain Control Using the Ring of Earth

My guide said the Ring of Earth was for physical re-creation and pain control, and that it would also help control addiction and seduction! He suggested physical locations for the circuit, and I picked out the corresponding acupuncture points.

He also said that this ring was useful to establish a magnetic contact with the earth, and that it would help patients overcome phobias; skin disorders; and seductions such as drug addiction, illusion, and possession. In addition, it would assist in redesigning the physical body. The Ring of Earth would also be useful for people with cerebral palsy, confusion, and physical pain.

I was also told that when the Ring of Earth is used with the Ring of Crystal, it would be beneficial for patients with multiple sclerosis, ALS, and Parkinson's disease. My angelic guide said that both the Ring of Earth and Ring of Crystal were needed for these neurological disorders. Parenthetically he stated that, "with seduction, the kidneys, liver, and sexual organs are at risk." I am not certain that this has any relation to the neurological problems!

The Ring of Earth—Circuit Points in the Body

- **Kidney 1** (Stimulate or apply Earth Bliss on the soles of the feet. Run a finger below the big bone of the long bone of the big toe into the space at the bottom of the head of the long bone of the second toe.)

- **Bladder 60** (Stimulate or apply Earth Bliss behind the outsides of the ankle bones, in that space between the anklebones and Achilles tendons.)

- **Bladder 54** (Stimulate or apply Earth Bliss directly behind the knees in the center.)

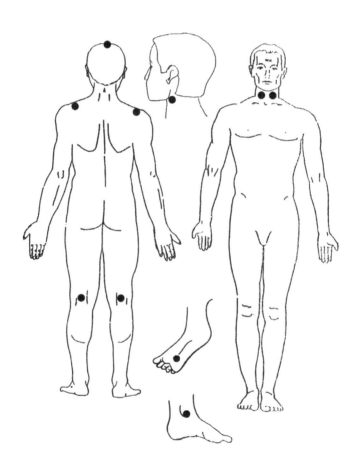

- **Large Intestine 16** (Stimulate or apply Earth Bliss to the point you find when you run your fingers behind the collarbones toward the shoulders as far as you can go, in the muscles just medial to the bones of the shoulders.)

- **Stomach 9** (Run your fingers along the throat from the top of where the Adam's apple is for men to that space before you come to the muscles. *Do not tap or massage this point!* Pinch the skin there and twist vigorously! Or apply Earth Bliss.)

- **Small Intestine 17** (Move your fingers out to grab the front of the muscle that is just beyond the S9 point (directly above) and pinch the front edges of the muscles. Or apply Earth Bliss.)

- **Governing Vessel 20** (Stimulate or apply Earth Bliss to the point on the top center of the skull, up from the ears.)

Results with Use of the Ring of Earth

I discovered that stimulation with the same human GHz frequencies raises calcitonin, which is the thyroid-produced hormone that helps maintain bone integrity (reduces osteoporosis). Calcitonin is also 40 to 60 times as powerful as morphine for pain relief.

As such, I have seen it work so well sometimes that it is the most powerful pain reliever I have ever found. The essential oil blend Earth Bliss works well to activate this ring, and it just takes a few seconds to apply.

I have found that individuals who have a daytime temperature of less than 98.6°F when it's taken orally may need to take iodine and stimulate the Ring of Fire to regenerate thyroid function in order for activation of the Ring of Earth to work. It also does help reverse osteoporosis.

A 45-year-old man who had suffered severe pain following a spinal injury obtained almost total relief of his pain the first time he stimulated the Ring of Earth. I know that Earth Bliss activates calcitonin, so I fully expect to receive many more similar reports of pain relief with these essential oils.

Reducing Free Radicals with the Ring of Crystal

The final ring, Crystal, came to me almost five years after the original Ring of Fire. As with the times before, my angelic guide provided me with the physical locations, and I chose the points. Through that process, the 13 points of the Ring of Crystal materialized.

My guide said that this circuit "regulates the overall energetic system and assists in regeneration." But once again, I was slow in intuiting the neurochemistry . . . but then it came to me suddenly. I knew it had to be reduction of free radicals, since these by-products of excess oxidation tend to destroy cell walls.

I already knew how important it is to keep free radicals in the body at a minimal level, and was excited at the potential that the Ring of Crystal could deliver. All our cells reproduce within a seven-year cycle, but they need a healthy place to grow. There is little point in the rebirth of healthy baby cells if they are only born into an unhealthy bath of free radicals! In such a toxic environment, these poor new cells don't have a chance and end up being reproduced, as they're already wrinkled and worn. I expected that the Ring of Crystal could help clean up this messy situation that's caused by too many free radicals, and so it did—an amazing 85 percent reduction in free radicals!

The Ring of Crystal—Circuit Points in the Body

- **Spleen 4** (Run your fingers back along the long bones of the big toe until you reach a joint on the inside of the feet. Wiggle your toes, and you will know you are on the joint; stimulate or apply Crystal Bliss.)

- **Gallbladder 30.5** (Standing, put your long fingers on the bottom of your buttocks muscles, and run the thumbs out halfway from back to front of the thighs. You should be right on the center of the femurs, the long bones of the thighs; stimulate or apply Crystal Bliss there.)

- **Conception Vessel 8.5** (Stimulate or apply Crystal Bliss a half inch directly above your belly button.)

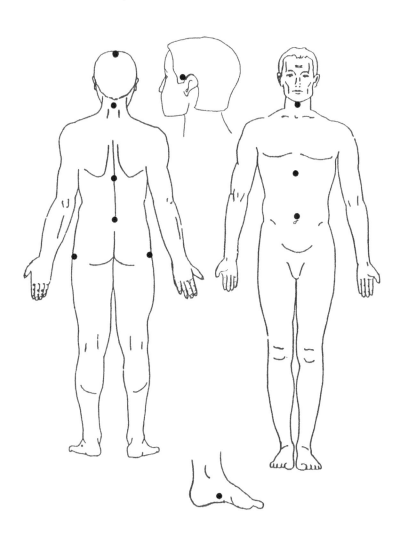

- **Governing Vessel 4.5** (Stimulate or apply Crystal Bliss directly behind Conception Vessel 8.5 over the center of the spine.)

- **Conception Vessel 14.5** (Stimulate or apply Crystal Bliss over the center of the bottom of the breastbone.)

- **Governing Vessel 7.5** (Stimulate or apply Crystal Bliss directly behind Conception Vessel 14.5 over the center of the spine.)

- **Conception Vessel 23** (This point is directly above the top of where the Adam's apple is located for men. *Do not tap here.* Pinch the skin and twist vigorously, or apply Crystal Bliss.)

- **Governing Vessel 14.4** (Stimulate or apply Crystal Bliss directly behind Conception Vessel 23, described just above, but this time in the center of your spine.)

- **Gallbladder 7** (Stimulate or apply Crystal Bliss bilaterally at the space on your scalp where the front of the ears joins the scalp.)

- **Governing Vessel 20** (Stimulate or apply Crystal Bliss to the point that is on the top center of the skull, up from the ears.)

Results with Use of the Ring of Crystal

I found that daily stimulation of the Ring of Crystal with GHz leads to 85 percent reduction in free radicals within three to five days—which is by far the best decrease in free radicals of anything I have seen or found.

Even more exciting, we now have 12 months' worth of follow-up data showing that Crystal Bliss essential oil blend reduces free radicals by 80 percent in the long term! I don't know of *anything* that is as effective as the Ring of Crystal for reducing free radicals. Some strong fruit concentrates reduce free radicals by 43 percent, and there is no evidence that the otherwise beneficial antioxidant supplements actually reduce free-radical output in the urine. Incidentally, you can purchase test kits called Oxidata online for the malondialdehyde measurement. Malondialdehyde is the breakdown product of free-radical destruction of cell walls, which are made of fat. That fat becomes a waste product excreted in the urine.

This brings us full circle to the connection to true longevity! Through stimulation of the Ring of Crystal, I could see that free radicals were lowered by 85 percent within three days, and I suddenly knew that if we stimulated the Rings of Fire, Earth, and Crystal in people who otherwise have good health habits, we should live an average of 140 years! This is truly the fountain of youth for the conscientious person—delivered in three easy-to-activate circuits.

Reviewing Activation Methods for the Sacred Rings

Before closing this chapter then, I want to remind you that these five rings can be activated in a number of ways. First, if you have invested already in your own Shealy PainPro, you can use this small device to electrically stimulate the points on your body that correspond to the circuits for that specific ring. Sadly, though, because most people did not want to spend the time to use this device—and because of the tedious U.S. Food and Drug Administration (FDA) requirements each year—I stopped manufacturing the Shealy PainPro as of December 2012. (*Tedious* would be the kindest way I could describe the FDA.)

But don't worry if you haven't got a Shealy PainPro. The second activation method is easier anyway: You can activate these rings by listening to one of my CD recordings that guides you in using your own mind to release the healing power of each ring.

The third and fourth activation methods that you might consider are a moderate massage of these circuit points or tapping them to release their power. These methods each take practice but can be quite effective for some individuals.

The fifth method is to use one of my five essential oil blends, which many patients find to be the quickest and easiest way to activate these circuits, namely Fire Bliss, Air Bliss, Earth Bliss, Water Bliss, and Crystal Bliss. Our offices in Missouri fill online and phone orders every day for these oils and other supplements that people find helpful in maintaining optimum health. This approach is now called *transcutaneous acupuncture,* a name I have found that is acceptable to physicians.

Coming Soon—The Ring of Life

Recently, I was very happy to receive initial details about a sixth circuit called the Ring of Life, and, as of this writing, its specific oil appears to be the strongest yet in affecting mood and potentially reducing the stress response. But for now, you'll just have to stay tuned on that matter.

At this point, it is a good time to return to our discussion of conscientiousness, because I'd like to share with you a number of life-changing lessons in spiritual healing and boosting conscientiousness that have truly transformed my own life.

CHAPTER EIGHT

LESSONS LEARNED AS STUDENT, TEACHER, AND MENTOR

In my junior year of medical school, I had to take a course in psychiatry. It was the worst class of my entire life! To this day, I have never experienced such incompetent teaching.

Among other oddities, we spent 12 weeks trying to answer Dr. Cohen's question "What is disease?" Finally, one of my classmates asked, "Dr. Cohen, if we ever answer 'What is disease?' to your satisfaction, what the hell are you going to do with it?" The whole class broke up laughing, and with that, he dismissed us in complete frustration.

Then we had a ridiculous final exam. I remember only one question: "List five qualities of a good psychiatrist." I wrote "Crazy as hell" five times!

Afterward, I was called to a meeting with several of the faculty, where they threatened to flunk me. I replied, "Do you want me in this stinking class again next year?" Thank God they saw the light and decided to pass me to avoid my threat!

It turns out that I never really did find a good reason for psychiatry to exist in this world—I know without a shadow of a doubt that it does more harm than good. And I surely did not need to take that course in psychiatry to be able to figure out the answer to Cohen's burning question "What is disease?"

As I mentioned earlier, when I was a young neurosurgeon, I came to the conclusion that disease and illness in the human body are caused by the interaction of the four main fields of stress: chemical, physical, electromagnetic, and emotional. Any kind of imbalance between these fields can cause disease.

Over the years, as I delved deeper into holistic and alternative healing therapies, I have revised my thinking to include the dangerous state of our health when we have an imbalance or friction between our thoughts and our souls. Whenever our thinking is not congruent with our soul's highest purpose, this can cause a state of *not* being at ease (also known as *dis-ease*), which manifests most often in our world as depression and anxiety; and, of course, these two dominant emotional issues are the foundations for an unlimited number of physical and biochemical disorders.

The Seeds of Our Belief Systems

So if our thoughts and belief systems are so critical to our well-being, where do they come from in the first place? From our earlier chapters, remember that our perspective of the world begins at conception and birth, and has a great deal to do with how we are nurtured and loved (or not) along the way.

I would say that our worldview and daily thoughts are also influenced by our teachers—and I use this term *teachers* broadly to describe all the people and the systems in our lives that have an impact on the way we see the world. To illustrate this, I'd like to describe some of my own major influences and lessons, starting with the most critical for all of us—our own parents, who are our first teachers.

As I've mentioned within this text, I believe that we have a choice about what we come into this life to learn. This means that we have the opportunity to choose the parents who can give us the right challenges in order to develop strong character and abilities.

My mother died exactly one month after her 97th birthday, and I could write a book about either her or my father. But the bottom line is that they were both perfect for me. As parents, they were supportive, nurturing, and encouraging. They taught me moral boundaries and provided me with virtually unlimited opportunities to explore my broad interests in school and in life.

Lessons Learned from My Father

My father was a successful businessman who left school at age ten when his father died. Dad became a butcher in a grocery store, and eventually he owned two grocery stores, a freezer locker, and a 600-acre farm. He even offered me a 7,000-acre farm with a colonial home if I would go to agriculture school instead of medical school, because he thought it would be less stressful.

But when I said no, that was the end of it. As much as he was concerned for my well-being, I was free to make my own decision—except for playing football.

Not all of my father's decisions were easy for him, nor were they all easy for me to accept. He stood his ground when his conscious mind and his common sense strongly told him to do so, even if I didn't like it. For example, my father loved the high school football team; he rarely missed a game. But when I wanted to go out for football, he refused to give me permission. He said that he did not want me to get hurt; he wanted to protect my brain and spine.

That was hard for me as a teenager to take, since of course I felt invincible. Once I became a neurosurgeon, however, I fully understood his position and discouraged my own boys from playing the sport. Incidentally, my close friend Henry Rucker chastised me when our son Brock was in eighth grade and wanted to try out for his school team. I reluctantly gave in, but once Brock injured his knee I refused to give him further permission to play—and his knee has been a lifelong problem for him. Like my father, I should have gone with the gut feelings I had in the first place.

In the fall of 1954, my father had his first heart attack. After he recovered, he came to the hospital at Duke University for an evaluation. I pleaded with him to quit smoking, but he replied, "I'd rather die than quit smoking."

From my point of view, this was my father's only problem—the fact that he smoked. During the last 15 years or so of his life he was very active in the Shriners and on the divan, on the way to be grand potentate when he died. (The Shriners are part of the Masonic order and are best known for their children's hospitals where neurological and orthopedic problems are treated. In each chapter of Shriners there is a leadership path in which one progresses up the ladder—or divan—to beome the Grand Potentate, or leader.) In his last few years of life, my father had angina decubitus. As a physician, I knew it was only a matter of time.

Dad died in 1962 from his third heart attack at the age of 53. I was only 29 years old, which was far too young to lose my father. From my point of view, he committed suicide by smoking, and I felt his loss deeply.

Then in 1994, he visited me from the other side with a message. He said, "I'm tired of your saying that I committed suicide. My life contract with you was to die at 53. I gave you an example of someone you would consider weak willed so that you could make the choice. You came into this life saying you wanted a strong will. You have a very strong-willed mother."

His message was so clear and chilling, but I knew it was from him and these were his true words. I took the opportunity to ask him, "You've been dead for over 30 years. Why didn't you tell me this earlier?"

His reply: "You weren't ready to hear it." I probably wasn't. But I am glad now to know the truth, and it makes sense to me.

Lessons Learned from My Mother

You know what? My father was right when he described my mother as very strong willed. Now that I think about it, she learned her lessons in strength and self-reliance from her own parents. She had a saintly mother herself (my maternal grandmother), but also an incredibly obnoxious father (my maternal grandfather). I'm not kidding—he was a mean SOB, and Mom couldn't get out of that house soon enough.

She left home at age 16 to marry my father, who was only 19. But my mother overcame the influences of her dad. She learned from him what kind of a parent she did *not* want to be, and instead chose to emulate her strong and self-sufficient mother.

My mother had many skills. She was quite bright and wise about investments; if she had been born 50 or 100 years later, quite likely she would have been a highly successful businessperson. But as with most women of her time, she was expected to stay at home. Even still, she took on every task with conscientiousness and purpose.

My mom loved children and even ran a day care for a number of years. She also adored Chihuahuas, which are virtually the only dogs that I don't like. They remind me of barking rats. Fortunately, no Chihuahuas lived in our house during my childhood. We had real dogs! And I still do—a young German shepherd and an older blue Australian cattle dog that both love the farm.

My mother was a compulsive housekeeper and a terrific gardener. When I turned 12, she encouraged me to take over the family vegetable garden, which had generally been maintained by her most of the time. I grew not only a variety of vegetables, but also many flowers.

I know that I got my own conscientiousness from my mother, and I developed a very strong work ethic thanks to both of my parents. I still love growing vegetables and flowers, and I still grow as much of my own food as I possibly can, enjoying crops, meat, and eggs from our farm.

Another fond memory of lessons from childhood was when I joined the Boy Scouts at age 12, just before my 13th birthday. My scoutmaster, James Sheeley, lived just a block away and became essentially a surrogate father to me. He had a small photography studio in his backyard, and I learned to develop, enlarge, and crop images from old-fashioned film. I spent many hours working in his studio. Because of the slight spelling difference of our last names, we decided we were, perhaps, 42nd cousins. I will never forget him as a strong role model, one of many father figures in my life.

Lessons Learned from My Sister

My older sister was born when my mother was 18, and I was born two years and eight months after my sister. During her pregnancy with me, Mom developed hyperthyroidism. She weighed only 75 pounds when I was born! Frail but coping, on one or two occasions my mother apparently turned her attention to taking care of me without adequately satisfying my sister's need for nurturing, and within six months my sister became depressed and overweight.

When I was four, I overheard her say to our mother that she had abandoned her when I was born. My mother strongly denied that she had done this, but it did not matter what the final truth was. My sister perceived that she was abandoned, and I believe she carried that hurt her whole life.

The impact of my sister's belief system did not hit me until much later in my life; in fact, it was years after her death before I knew the truth about it.

During our years growing up, I knew she resented me. She had a tough life, but I had everything come easy to me—at least that's the way she would tell it. Just as an example, I remember the June that my sister graduated from high school. On commencement day, just before the graduation exercise, class honors were given out. I was as stunned as anyone when they called me to the stage to receive five honors for best in the class in Latin, history, Spanish, and so on. My sister was mortified and furious that I upstaged her on her own graduation day. To her, it was just one more situation where she was slighted.

Although she claimed that our mother had abandoned her, my sister did not leave home until she was 30, when she got married. Regretfully, she continued to struggle with her weight, and she died from complications of obesity and diabetes at age 58 in 1988.

Incidentally, six years after her death her spirit also visited me from the other side. She told me, "I just wanted you to know it wasn't you. I learned the path of the heart from the shadow side." I asked her, "And what is my path?" She replied, "To learn the path of the heart from the light side." It was a moment of clarity that I will never forget. I immediately knew that, despite my tremendous love and compassion for other people, I never allowed anyone to get close to me. Her message opened up the floodgates for me, and from that point on I had my heart open in both directions—being able to love fully and to be loved, and to express both pure joy and deep sadness.

From That Point of Kundalini Awakening

The experience of hearing my sister's message in 1994 seemed to cause a sudden opening of my heart chakra, and it felt like one of the greatest, most painful heart experiences I've ever had. But now I can cry much more easily—expressing emotions during joyful and sad times.

Before it happened to me, I had heard about this kind of Kundalini awakening, a kind of spiritual breakthrough. The word *Kundalini* is the ancient Sanskrit name for the primal life force that animates all living entities. It operates unconsciously in our bodies and minds until awakened, initiating a much greater opportunity for spiritual growth, enlightenment, and the advancement of one's own personal evolution in a dramatic way. I certainly found that I was far more open to divine inspiration after this incident.

A couple of weeks later, in 1994, I was at Findhorn in northern Scotland, which is a beautiful location and a world-renowned center for spiritual growth and organic farming. Caroline Myss and I were there to give a workshop together. With my new open heart, I felt sad about being away from my wife. As I walked along the beach covered with smooth rocks, suddenly, in the middle of this rocky sand, a heart-shaped white stone with a red streak down the center popped out at me, almost jumping into my hand. I took it as a sign of my new awakening, and I still treasure it today.

Other Lessons Learned While Traveling with Caroline Myss

I have been a willing teacher but also a student—I learn from my patients, my colleagues, my family, and from everyone with whom I connect.

My friend Caroline reminds me often that my attempt to unconditionally love will attract every obnoxious person possible in order to provide an opportunity to practice! This has been true in my life. I've had some truly dreadful lessons, but also many loving ones. Thus, I especially bless my most intimate family, for they make it easy for me to practice loving them as unconditionally as possible.

One of the most entertaining times Caroline and I had together was in the early 1990s when we traveled to Holland to give a conference presentation to 800 health and holistic practitioners at a meeting being held in The Hague. A very proper and officious Dutch woman was in charge of organizing the conference, and she picked us up at the airport, very happy that we had arrived on time. We could tell that she was a no-nonsense sort of woman, highly conscientious—everything was planned down to the minute.

While she was making small talk with Caroline and me during the car ride on the way to the meeting, she asked us what we would be speaking about in our presentation. I said off the cuff, "Oh, I don't know. We'll probably just wing it as we usually do."

Caroline and I just laughed, but the woman in charge gasped and almost drove off the road! She was obviously shocked that these two North American experts had arrived with no preparation to present at her highly organized and prestigious conference. We quickly reassured her that we had it all under control, but we could tell she was still pretty nervous for the rest of the long drive.

As I recall, the meeting itself went amazingly well, as usual. Caroline and I had a lot of experience co-presenting, and we would always tailor our commentary to the interests of those in the room. It turned out that at this particular conference she and I would get the chance to laugh some more and be reminded of something very valuable at the same time.

The Healing Power of Laughter

Among the attendees we thoroughly enjoyed hearing was a Dutch dermatologist who gave a spirited demonstration of laughing-meditation techniques. The session reminded me of the power of laughter to heal, and this experience prompted me to conduct my own study.

We had subjects who were experiencing pain watch old Abbott and Costello movies, and we found that when they enjoyed periods of sustained laughter, their brains and bodies released neurochemicals called beta-endorphins that induce feelings of well-being. Our own study of laughter was congruent with the dermatologist's assertion—that laughter is effective in helping the body manage pain.

This harkened me back to an experiment I had heard about in the 1970s that was done by Norman Cousins, a celebrated writer and editor for the *Saturday Review*. Cousins gave a personal account of his own battle with disease and recovery in his book *Anatomy of an Illness,* which detailed how he left the hospital and checked into a hotel to pursue an alternative treatment.

The treatment that he chose centered on intravenous delivery of vitamin C coupled with daily doses of belly laughter from watching old movies and funny videos. As Cousins so famously documented in his book, this course of treatment was successful!

I always loved traveling with Caroline Myss. She is a good example of being both a student and a teacher to me. She has very graciously stated in print, "I was more than lucky in finding Norm as my mentor; I was blessed. And this I know to be true above all else—you cannot walk into the territory of the soul unescorted. A mentor is essential."

I am very thankful to Caroline and my own teachers and mentors in all areas of life, but especially in the medical, holistic, and spiritual fields of study. Their guidance has been absolutely essential to my development. I have had so many amazing teachers in school and in life, that I will share just a few examples to give you an idea of the dynamics involved.

Lessons Learned from Dr. Talmage Peele

One of my most important discoveries during medical school was my love of neuroanatomy. Most students dislike it, but to me it's the most exciting anatomy of all. Dr. Talmage Peele was the neuroanatomy professor and was just writing his textbook on the subject while I was there, so I volunteered to help proofread it. By the end of that year, we had become lifelong friends. Like James Sheeley, he was like a surrogate father to me.

Since I had not yet finished my undergraduate degree, I wanted to get my bachelor of science in medicine, a degree that Duke offered to medical students who did research and a thesis. I chose to work on the anatomy and physiology of the amygdaloid nucleus (also called *amygdala*) of cats. After each of the first three years of medical school, I spent three months doing research in Dr. Peele's lab, which was located in the room immediately adjacent to his office. It was a great place to hang out, and he had a delightful sense of humor about life in general.

Talmage also had a small circle of faculty friends who met frequently, and they invited me to dinner quite often. They introduced me to some rather exotic, gourmet dishes, such as chocolate-covered grasshoppers. As I had promised my father, I did not drink alcohol until my 21st birthday, which was on December 4, 1953. That was when Talmage introduced me to his favorite Usher's Green Stripe scotch. Even after medical school,

I very often sought and received mentoring from Talmage, who always called me "Junior."

I remember well that my first published paper was on the physiology of the amygdala of the cat—which are small nuclei located deep within the temporal lobe of the brain. I had a few findings that were not previously known about this essential emotional center, and Talmage was proud of me, always supportive. Virtually all my experiences learned while doing research in his lab proved invaluable to my later work when I developed dorsal column stimulation, which I perfected first on cats.

Some Lessons Come Easy, Some Hard

After my one-year internship in internal medicine, I had to take a year in general surgery as an assistant resident. Only two places in the country would allow that—Boston City Hospital and Barnes-Jewish Hospital in St. Louis. I needed a reference from Dr. Eugene Stead, Jr., who was chair of medicine at Duke, and told him my choices. He replied, "Choose one. I will write you *one* recommendation." I chose Barnes.

I learned later that Gene wrote to Dr. Carl Moyer at Barnes-Jewish Hospital, which is located near the campus of Washington University in St. Louis, "Dear Carl: Take him." Dr. Moyer was my reason for choosing Barnes. He is one of the three greatest teachers of my life, along with Talmage Peele and Gene Stead.

Dr. Moyer held teaching rounds at 2 P.M. on Saturdays, and the room was always packed. St. Louis that year was the hottest summer of my life. In staff barracks, which was a non-air-conditioned building where I lived, it was sometimes 100°F at midnight. I chose rotations in general surgery: neurosurgery; orthopedics; and chest surgery, and each department was excellent.

The next step was to select a neurosurgery program, and the top ones in the country at the time were Duke, Barnes, and Mass General. I was accepted into all three programs, but I chose Mass General, certainly another one of the most critical decisions of my life. Dr. Henry Schwartz at Barnes was known as "Black Henry" because of his temper, but he was a superb surgeon. His temper in the operating room was legendary.

On one occasion, Schwartz hit me in the abdomen with his elbow so hard that I almost passed out. His comment was, "Damn you. Don't breathe so hard." When working on a patient who had a high cervical cordotomy under local anesthesia, he screamed, "Damn you! Be still or I will cut your damned head off."

Once Schwartz even stabbed my hand with a scalpel. And he ordered the chief resident, Dr. Herbert Lourie, one of the best surgeons and personalities I ever knew, out of the operating room. I think I lost several heartbeats at the thought of being the only one left with Schwartz in the OR, and I held my breath to see what would happen next.

Fortunately, Herb replied, "Dr. Schwartz, I have not done anything to be thrown out of the operating room." And Black Henry the bully was silent for the rest of the case.

Halfway through my rotation at Barnes, I went to Boston for an interview. Afterward, I told Dr. Schwartz that I had chosen to go to Mass General for my neurosurgery training. He snarled at me and replied, "You've made the wrong choice." He never spoke to me during the last six weeks of my neurosurgery rotation, which I would say was a blessing.

Making the Right Decisions

At each turn, I relied on my own sense of conscientiousness to make the best decisions for my life, and I was very thankful for the guidance of my mentors. Given time and perspective, I also appreciated some of the nasty encounters as well, because I know that they were there to help me build a stronger character in the long run. My career path reflected steady advancement while we were living in Wisconsin, but keeping things steady at the farm became less straightforward.

My biggest issue was that our real-estate taxes increased by 600 percent between 1975 and 1980. I was convinced that we could no longer afford to live on our farm, and so my search for an alternative location became intense. We looked primarily at Virginia, North Carolina, and Missouri. Of the three, Missouri had the 49th lowest taxes per capita, so we set our sights on making the "Show-Me" state our new home.

I didn't want to live near a large city like St. Louis or Kansas City, so Springfield looked like it was the best option. During the weekend of Easter 1981, we made our second trip there and decided that it was best for us, even though we didn't know anyone in the area.

The Monday after Easter, I received a phone call out of the blue from Jon Ames, who was vice president of the St. John's Regional Medical Center (recently changed to Mercy Hospital) in Springfield. He said that they wanted a pain center and were told repeatedly to contact me for advice. He had no idea about our plans to move, so he was a bit shocked when I answered him cheerfully, "How would you like to have mine?" It took only a few more visits to confirm the arrangement, and after that Chardy and I made the move with three children, the horses, and the pain clinic. I feel that the universe meant for us to make this move, since it worked out seamlessly in the end.

Coinciding with the move to Springfield, I set up a nonprofit 501(c)(3) corporation, Holos Institutes of Health, Inc., for the purpose of education, research, and clinical services in the field of holistic medicine and health. My new pain clinic at St. John's was then converted into a division of Holos Institutes. This arrangement made it much easier to obtain grants and tax-deductible donations and certainly was an excellent strategic move all the way around.

Advancing the Study of Holistic Medicine

In the mid-1990s, a Dutch businessman who was a friend of Caroline Myss and mine, flew over to see us and spent several days pushing us to do more research in the field of medical intuition and the broader field of holistic medicine. I finally said, "Fred, we would need a $50 million endowment to do what needs to be done."

Since this was not an option, the only way I could see us doing the kind of research he was talking about was to start a graduate program where doctoral students would do research as part of their dissertation. Since I had just served on the faculty committee that counseled students at Greenwich University, which, at the time, was a distance-learning institution in Hawaii, I wrote to the president there and asked about the possibility of having a doctoral program in energy medicine. He was delighted. They created the program, and it thrived—100 students enrolled the first two years.

Unfortunately, just a few years later, Greenwich University was sold to an Australian who moved the university to Norfolk Island in the Pacific Ocean, located between Australia and New Zealand. The administration changed, and with the school now located on the other side of the world, it became obvious that we needed to create an American school.

We approached the Missouri Department of Higher Education and learned that they would never approve a new doctoral program unless it originated in an already accredited university or if it was run by a seminary. So it was in 2000 that we decided to create Holos University Graduate Seminary (HUGS), a graduate school offering doctoral degrees in spiritual healing and energy medicine. Initially, we set it up so that the seminary was run by the International Science of Mind Church for Spiritual Healing— the church that was originally created in 1973 by Henry Rucker and me.

I had previous experience serving on the faculty of The School of Professional Psychology at Forest Institute, so I knew that the accrediting body did not like presidents over the age of 65. We were pushing it since I was already 68 when we set it up, so from the beginning I planned to serve as president only until age 75. I hoped that I would be with HUGS long enough to help it eventually become nationally accredited. Many of our initial students came over from the Greenwich program, which meant that our first graduation took place in the spring of 2001.

The timing of it all worked out quite well, because I had been looking to move out of the city of Springfield for a while, having found that the background electromagnetic "smog" was very high in the city—two and a half to three milligauss. So I sold the clinic in town and built a facility on two acres of our land located at the entrance to our farm.

The facility was finished in the spring of 2003 and became the new home of Holos Institutes of Health, Inc., a place dedicated to research, education, and clinical services, and to which we donated the land itself. As was our plan, we also housed the seminary there until my retirement in the summer of 2008, and then it moved to Unity Village just southeast of Kansas City, Missouri, where we now conduct residency classes.

My Teaching Focus at Holos University
Graduate Seminary

Over the years, I have had several specialties that I have taught within HUGS, including holistic theology, medical intuition, modern mysticism, and clinical applications of energy medicine. The teaching was done by way of classroom intensives, each lasting for a total of two to five days of lectures and demonstrations, with homework assignments and papers to be written. Up until my retirement, I was also the chair overseeing many dissertation projects.

I still enjoy getting back into the classroom when I can. Last year, for example, Caroline and I taught a course on mysticism and health. My premise for this course began with the assertion that mysticism is the *search* for God and religion is the *fight* for God. Holistic theology then looks at the broader field of world religions, focusing on the conflicts as well as the few universal principles across the board. It also examines the inconsistencies in the Bible and the innumerable changes to this text through the centuries.

I have read and studied just about every philosophical, spiritual, and religious theory along my way, and today I consider myself to be a pantheistic Buddhist. Pantheism is the belief that everything is composed of an all-encompassing God, and that the universe (or nature) is identical with divinity. So I don't believe in a personal or anthropomorphic god.

I feel most closely aligned to Buddhism because, in and of itself, it is not a religion, but a philosophy and a way of life. There were no gods in Buddhism in the strictest sense; the teachings of Buddha, in the beginning, were about how to think, act, and function in order to attain enlightenment.

Holos University Graduate Seminary continues its work based in Kansas City, fully accredited by the New Thought Accreditation Commission, which is the amalgamation of the Unity Church, the Church of Religious Science, and the Church of Divine Science. Full details are at www.holosuniversity.org.

Finding Someone to Take Over My Work

In 1980, during what were to be my last 18 months in La Crosse, Wisconsin, before we moved to Missouri, I met a family-practice resident named Roger Cady, whom I mentioned in the previous chapter. I hoped that Roger would join me at the clinic when he finished his residency, but instead he wanted the experience of a family practice first. Fortunately, by 1985 Roger was ready to join me, and he and his family agreed to move to the Springfield, Missouri, area, which was our new base.

Shortly after he arrived, I made what may have been a tactical error. I was invited to present some of my pain work at a national meeting in San Diego. Tired from all the travel, I asked Roger to give the talk for me. As a result, GlaxoSmithKline asked Roger to be part of the clinical research on sumatriptan, a new drug for migraine treatment. In the end, our clinic treated more patients with this new drug than any other clinic in the study.

Personally, I never wanted to do clinical drug research, as all drugs have inherent risks in the form of rather innocent-sounding side effects, which are really complications. I'm sure that if I had given the talk and they had asked me, I would not have agreed.

On the other hand, I was delighted that Roger had a unique new interest. I was blessed to have him with me for ten years, and hoped he would someday take over the clinic. However, toward the end of that time, it became clear that he felt he would always be in my shadow. Since he was becoming quite popular and well respected as a headache researcher and speaker, he left my clinic in 1995 and founded the Headache Care Center. He remains at the forefront in that field, and we are still the best of friends.

Although I found a few part-time physicians to help me with the clinic once Roger left, it was difficult to find the one individual who I needed to take over. I required someone with the right personality to assume the demanding task of handling difficult invalids with chronic pain and depression.

Eventually, a perfect possibility arrived: the daughter of one of my previous colleagues at the Gundersen Clinic. Unfortunately, though, she died of acute Addison's disease in less than a year. I realized when I looked through my files that I had interviewed 100 physicians over the course of the years and not found the right one. I therefore decided to close the clinic in 2003 and restrict myself to research.

Fast-forward almost ten years later, and I still had it in my heart and mind that I wanted to advance my current research work, particularly the field of conscientious psychology, which has become my consuming passion. As I continued to look around for the best way to accomplish this during these past few years, I am very happy to say that I figured it out! The solution and my new intended directions are next, as I sum up this book and begin plans for the next one.

ᴖᴖᴖ ᴖᴖᴖ

CHAPTER NINE

THE FUTURE OF CONSCIENTIOUS PSYCHOLOGY

When I decided to spend the rest of my life studying, teaching, and motivating others toward conscientiousness, I wondered how best to do this. Less conscientious people might have long since given up their dream after reaching 78 years of age and not finding someone suitable to take on this challenge. However, I am pleased to say that I found a way to do it, and we are on our way!

My idea was to establish a research chair in conscientious psychology, and I approached Missouri State University (MSU) about it. I suggested that I would like to set up an endowment to the university in order to establish and fund this research position. I decided to call it the Mary-Charlotte Bayles Shealy Chair of Conscientious Psychology, so named for the most conscientious person I have known, Chardy Shealy, my late wife of 52 years. The research chair would be housed at MSU, but his or her work would also be a major focus for the Holos Building of my 501(c)(3) organization, the Holos Institutes of Health.

My relationship with both the agriculture and psychology departments at MSU has been gratifyingly cooperative, and I have been invited by the search committee for the chair to work with them to choose that person, hopefully by the time this book is published.

Chardy's death in 2011 was the impetus to set this up in her memory, an endowment made possible through the donation of our farm to the university. My donation is 256 acres of land; the animals; all the buildings, including the 11,000-square-foot health research conference center that was completed in 2003; and a substantial additional financial gift.

I asked our three children if they had an interest in the farm, and since they did not, I am quite comfortable donating everything. I will live out my days in my home on the farm with a life-estate use of the house, as per our agreement.

MSU officially announced the endowment in January 2013 and unveiled their plans to have the William H. Darr School of Agriculture use the farm for hands-on student learning, which will include a beefalo production cattle ranch (beefalo is a hybrid between domestic cattle and buffalo). In addition, the health-research conference center, with its stunning chapel, has become a university-wide retreat center.

Coming to Terms with the End of a Conscientious Life

As I have said a few times, my wife, Mary-Charlotte, was not only conscientious, but also gifted in many other ways. In particular, she always had a deep and abiding love of horses and took up horseback riding early on in our married life. For her birthday in 1969, I gave her an Appaloosa gelding named Shadrick, and we earnestly began looking for the farm that we had wanted for so long.

We chose one in Welch Coulee—which is one of the beautiful valleys in that area of Wisconsin—with rolling hills and eventually 565 acres of land. Before long, Chardy and two friends developed a partnership, and we were breeding Appaloosas! There was no holding back my wife's love of horses, and she had a true gift in relating to these majestic animals. Throughout her career, she became known worldwide for her unique Success-Centered Riding and Training program, a therapeutic horse-riding program for adults.

Chardy and I lived perhaps the healthiest of lifestyles on our farms, first in Wisconsin and then in Missouri. Despite that, she also had a genetic predisposition to myelodysplasia—her father,

her grandmother, and an uncle all experienced similar problems. So even though we can control 75 percent of factors that impact health and longevity through conscientious living, when faced with the reality of our genetics (which control the other 25 percent), we can't always change the overall outcome.

I had been retired from HUGS for a few years, and was focused primarily on research, when I returned home from yet another workshop trip in 2010 to Chardy telling me that her heart was racing. I checked, and clearly she had a pulse of 120. The following day we got a chemistry and blood count panel done, and we learned that she had acute myelogenous leukemia (AML), which evolved from myelodysplasia.

I knew very little about AML before Chardy's diagnosis, and the following 13 months were a startling awakening. She refused the most radical therapy, which would have meant total destruction of her blood system with the hope that it could be coaxed back. Even if she had taken that route, the more traditional hematologist warned us that life expectancy would still be only about three months or less.

We sought further course of action and found a kind and enthusiastic hematologist in Bolivar, our county seat. He offered two less-toxic chemotherapies and gave us the success rate of each one. What we did not understand from the beginning was that his measure of success would have most likely given us only about three to six months.

It turned out both of these therapies failed, and even *he* gave up in October 2010. He was completely satisfied with our plan to use huge dosages of vitamin C, given through an IV two to three times a week, combined with a variety of other alternative approaches, including assistance from several healers and the prayers of hundreds.

Up until the Monday before her death, we fully expected Chardy to recover. That day she awoke and said, "I think we better go to the hospital." She did not return home to us.

I am most grateful to that small hospital for their superb care. The oncologist was pleased with himself, telling me that he thought her 13-month survival was great. That's when my heart sank even further, as I realized that he never believed she'd recover. Now I remain in recovery since her death in 2011, dealing with this crushing blow and a monumental loss that I still feel in my heart.

Life Continues with Each New Dawn

Notwithstanding all of this, the sun still rises every morning, and so do I. The farm comes alive at dawn, and I am up at five each day to exercise and feed the chickens.

It soothes my heart to take in the sweeping view that we have here of the rolling Missouri countryside, and I live to breathe in the fresh country air. Once the chores are done, I catch up on my reading, writing, and research, plus checking e-mails. A few hours later, when the rest of the country is just starting its day, I check in with the staff over at NOB (the building so named because it is the "New Office Building" on our property). This is where we process and fulfill online and phone orders for products through Shealy Wellness; it's always busy over there.

I sometimes see an occasional patient at the urging of a friend and at no charge, but I have not had a regular practice since 1999. On Thursdays, I drive 14 miles over to Springfield for my call-in radio show on KWTO, *Dr. Shealy's Wellness Hour*. This is a habit that I'm very happy to continue—I look forward to it each week, and I know the listeners do, too. I also have another two hours of call-in radio, when I join my friend Vincent Finelli on his *USA Prepares* show.

I've traveled most of my life, so I am no longer keen to be away all the time, but I do participate in about 18 or so meetings each year, and I occasionally do workshops on energy medicine or medical intuition. It's nice because I can just pick the things I like to do—there's no pressure to be everywhere at once the way it used to be. I am also doing a number of training workshops on transcutaneous acupuncture for health professionals.

But mostly I just do what I love, which is research. In fact, in addition to completing this book and continuing my own research on conscientious psychology, I am also studying insomnia and diabetic neuropathy. For the past ten years, my research was conducted at the Holos health research building that we built on our property. And I have agreed to write three more books immediately after this one.

A Unique Building Made for Research

The Holos building is a uniquely built structure with common rooms, offices, a boardroom/library, and a large multipurpose chapel on the main floor. Then there is another library downstairs, with a kitchen and various other rooms and devices that have been connected to my research efforts in holistic and alternative healing.

One of the unique gems of this health building is the chapel, complete with a built-in Navajo labyrinth; 20 specially lighted stained-glass hangings; a marble altar with inlays from the quarry from which the Taj Mahal was built; carvings and statues of Krishna, Tara, Buddha, and Shiva; and a magnificent mandala that was created for the great theologian Marcus Bach and given to me by his widow. There are also magnificent paintings of *Christ* by RoZelma Brown and *Into the Light* by Karla Brandt. The chapel is really the heart and soul of the building.

Downstairs there is a quartz room, which has four walls made from one ton of quartz crystal. For most people, sitting in this room quiets the idle chatter of the mind. We have a room with a vibratory bed set up with what looks like a jungle gym overhead. There are several speakers placed above the bed and ten actually in the bed that make the mattress vibrate. This is so patients can feel the music, which we've proven over the years has a much greater therapeutic effect than just hearing it.

In another room, there is a bed located over one ton of gold iodide crystals. Claude Swanson, Ph.D., a quantum physicist, says that this produces pure yin energy that is maximally relaxing. There is also a bed over one ton of mica crystal, which Claude says is pure yang energy, or maximally energizing. Another feature we added is a hot tub that is embedded in six tons of energizing mica crystal. And of course, there is a meditation grotto with a solid quartz bench.

Down the hall is another room with a wall covered with a large span of copper. In the early 1990s, I began experimenting on the effects of having individuals sit near the copper with a magnet placed over their heads. We found that it helped people release unfinished anger or depression, which gave them unique insights into their unresolved issues.

Releasing is much easier once we know what we're dealing with, and we saw many patients heal from their mental, emotional, and physical problems through the numerous therapeutic approaches we introduced them to. All these accessories make the Holos health building ideal for faculty meetings, retreats, and small conferences, which are increasingly used by MSU.

Honoring Those Who Came Before: Ambrose and Olga Worrall

The Holos building also houses a tribute to Ambrose and Olga Worrall, which I set up in honor of my dear friends and their roles as holistic pioneers. I began this quest in 1984 when I first recognized that Olga was becoming somewhat frail. I established a division of Holos Institutes of Health called the Ambrose and Olga Worrall Institute for Spiritual Healing.

I was so pleased that Olga was able to come for the formal inauguration, but unfortunately it was her last trip from Baltimore to see me. Her health deteriorated so rapidly that she died less than two years later.

I visited her a few months before her passing, but quickly learned that watching someone so close to me suffer was overwhelming for me. Before she died, Olga arranged to have Holos inherit much of her memorabilia, including her meditation bench and 15,000 testimonial letters from her healed patients. Later, I also received the wonderful painting of Ambrose and Olga, which had been a prominent feature in her living room, and another painting of Olga from earlier in her life.

The Healing Power of Copper Pyramids

Since divine insights can come at any time and in any number of ways, I was not too shocked one morning while jogging to suddenly have a vivid image of a copper pyramid on top of copper walls. When I got back to my room, I drew a sketch. About 36 hours later, my angelic guide suddenly came into my consciousness and asked me, "Norman, where do you think that image you received yesterday came from?"

I replied, "I thought it was mine."

He laughed and said, "I put it there. And you are to work on it."

On several other occasions, I discussed this concept with the same guide. He assured me that most of my intuitive hits were messages from him that came subliminally. How can I argue when these inspired innovations have helped improve the lives of thousands of patients and have given me 12 patents? I accept that they are the result of my spontaneous knowing of information sent from the divine.

Of course, when I returned home, I built the copper "room within a room" as he suggested—with the pyramid on top. I got permission from our institutional review board to treat 75 patients in this room while a Tesla coil was connected to the copper.

The results were outstanding. Not only did virtually all individuals report feelings of deep relaxation and peace by just sitting in the activated copper space of the pyramid, but 75 percent of them who had rheumatoid arthritis (who had failed conventional medicine) experienced marked improvement. We saw that 70 percent of the people with chronic lower-back pain improved, too, as did 70 percent of the depressed patients, who experienced a significant improvement in mood.

Using the same human DNA frequencies (54 to 78 billion cycles per second at 75 decibels of energy), we later demonstrated that individuals with diabetic neuropathy improved by 80 percent. In addition, 75 percent of those who were suffering with migraines improved.

The Telomere Connection to Longevity

If conscientiousness can help us live longer and more healthier lives, and our genes are good, what other things might sideline us on our way to living until, say, 110 or 120 years old? One thing I came across that seems to be a significant factor in aging is the reality of telomeres in our body.

Since becoming interested in this aspect of life, I am happy to say my research into telomeres still continues. Think of telomeres as little bookends at the ends of our chromosomes (a chromosome is a long strand of DNA). Telomeres keep chromosomes protected at the ends and also play an important role in cell division and reproduction.

We are born with telomeres in full size and strength, but they shrink by about 1 percent each year from birth onward, and the human body itself seems to be programmed to die at about 100 years of age. It simply wears out, and scientists feel part of this has to do with telomeres. You can think of them as getting shorter each time a cell divides, sort of like a pencil eraser that gets smaller each time it's used. Our cells stop replicating when telomeres get too short.

A few years ago, I developed a theory claiming that in order to live healthily up until 120 years of age or more, we would need to regenerate the telomeres in our bodies. This can be done by exposing ourselves to an electromagnetic field of 54 to 78 billion cycles per second at one-billionth of a watt per centimeter squared. I proved that it could be done using a Tesla coil attached to copper;

when exposed to this current, the telomeres stopped their natural decline and began to regenerate themselves at an average of 4.5 percent each year instead of shrinking by a percent. Mine have now grown almost 20 percent instead of shrinking the "expected" 6 percent.

For practical use, I decided to try putting a pure copper screen in the center layer of a mattress and scattering on top of that one pound of crushed sapphire crystal. This was put in between two one-inch pieces of polyfoam. I was partial to sapphire, because my guide had once told me that crushing and putting it over the heart would circumvent the need for bypass surgery. Using the energy in this way is really electrical homeopathy, and it is safe because it is 1,000 times lower than any risk level.

When people would lie on this mattress for 30 to 60 minutes a day or night, 70 percent of those tested experienced a regrowth of their telomeres at a rate of 4.5 percent per year. The results are fantastic, and so the project continues. In fact, with the benefit of transcutaneous acupuncture, I now have a number of individuals using Fire, Earth, and Crystal Bliss, which I intuitively believe will also regenerate telomeres.

Finding Your Ultimate Purpose

In December 2012, I turned 80. I did not expect to be here on my own, but life dealt me that card. However, I still get up with passion every day—my work is not "work," per se. It is joy; it is bliss. Even though I faced the hardest loss of my life when Chardy died, I did not give in to depression and sorrow. I may have the occasional low day, as we all do, but I continue to get up each morning and focus on my purpose.

For example, I feel a need to be on the radio each week—listeners count on me to return their e-mail questions and continue to cheer them on. My voice is known all over the Ozarks, and I know people find it comforting. Just about every time I walk into a store or public place around here, the minute I open my mouth to say anything, someone in line will turn and say, "Your voice! You sound just like Dr. Shealy on the radio." It makes them smile so brightly when I tell them that I *am* Dr. Shealy, and that makes me happy, too.

I am a very fortunate man. Each day I get to fulfill my lifelong dream, which is to help people heal and stay well. I am committed to keeping a positive attitude more than 90 percent of the time, and to be flexible enough to change quickly when necessary.

I have decided to do this 365 days a year, and I personally choose to keep moving and be productive until the day I die. It is my fervent desire to stay out of the pit of grief from the loss of the most important part of my life, Chardy.

I know I can do this—rise up each day—because I was grounded with outstanding nurturing from my parents, teachers, and wonderful friends. Plus, whenever I need a reminder, I have the Air Bliss essential oil blend and the Ring of Air to lift my spirits.

The Future of Conscientious Psychology

I see only tremendous potential for further research advances in the age-old field of energy medicine and through the newly endowed chair in conscientious psychology at MSU, which will be filled before the fall of 2014.

I believe that we have more than enough evidence for the benefits of conscientiousness; in my mind, conscientious psychology as a field of study should then focus on developing more proven tools for *increasing* self-esteem and conscientiousness. We need to extol the virtues of living this type of life and provide more practical tools and more education about what it entails; when we do, we will all be happier and healthier!

I hope that you will take the main lessons from this book into your own heart and soul. Find your purpose. Do it through conscientiousness. Even if you weren't nurtured as a child, you can be kind now and nurture yourself. If you need help to jump-start yourself out of depressive thoughts or anxiety, try Air Bliss and the other lifestyle changes that I've offered.

Collectively, the actions that I have described provide the essential foundation for living a purposeful, conscious, and conscientious life. Autogenic training is particularly powerful, and once you are eating well, sleeping soundly, and exercising five times a week, you will notice your energy level soar and your life improve. When you do good for yourself, you will have the energy to do good for others.

Remember, it is worth taking the effort to do these things each day; you are worth the effort! No one has to live in pain and depression. Take action, and you will thrive—you, too, will find your *Bliss!*

❧❧❧ ❧❧❧

APPENDIX

Provided by William A. Tiller, Ph.D.

Introduction to the Appendix by
C. Norman Shealy, M.D., Ph.D.

Since I'm quite comfortable with the field of parapsycholo-gy and psychics, I have been equally at home with many meta-physical concepts. When I met Dr. William Tiller in 1972, I was immediately impressed by his ability to convert metaphysics into physics and connect them with the greater concepts of multiple dimensions. For the past 40 years I have been blessed to read many of Bill's descriptions of interdimensional space. To a great extent, he correlates not only physics and metaphysics, but also religion and spirituality. From a practical point of view, those of us who live in the physical world are familiar with concepts such as spirit, soul, ghosts, angels, the etheric body, and so on.

A century ago, Einstein's theories took us from our concept of a three-dimensional world to one of four dimensions, with space-time representing the fourth dimension. Our concepts of space and time are related—thus, the theory of relativity—and even Ein-stein eventually agreed, reluctantly, that there is a fifth dimension.

But spiritual reality is not seen or measured in our fourth di-mension; therefore, there have to be further dimensions. In the past few decades, the influences of the mind and intention have also proven that thinking can impact every aspect of our world, from events to outcomes, the EEG, and even our genes! Epigenetics has emerged as one of the most exciting scientific fields, demonstrating that we can change the expression of many genes. Thus, the mind and emotions have *significant physical effects* upon our fourth-dimensional reality.

Acupuncture is an ancient art that has been unequivocally proven to have remarkable electrical, biochemical, and emotional benefits, even though it has no known physical anatomical structure. Thus, it is reasonable to consider acupuncture one of the interdimensional conduits. Now, with the use of the essential oils through transcutaneous acupuncture, another major connection has been proven. There is an interdimensional connection of the subtle etheric body with the physical body. I am most grateful to Dr. Tiller for his major contribution to the physics of intention and the interdimensional aspect of the five rings, as well as for allowing me to include his work here in this Appendix:

ᵕ ᵕ ᵕ

We are all souls and require a *physical body* to fully experience the distance-time domain! As humans, we wear our "biobodysuit"—which develops when we souls are born into nature's distance-time classroom—for the relatively short period of about 50 to 100 years, in space-time units, and then discard it when we leave this particular playpen of consciousness to return to higher-dimensional domains of reality.

Experience in this particular playpen allows us to (1) grow in *coherence,* and (2) develop our gifts of *intentionality.* In this way we can become what we were always intended to become: co-creators with our spiritual parents.

As a working hypothesis, I like to picture the soul self and its biobodysuit (the personality self) as illustrated in Figure 1[1]:

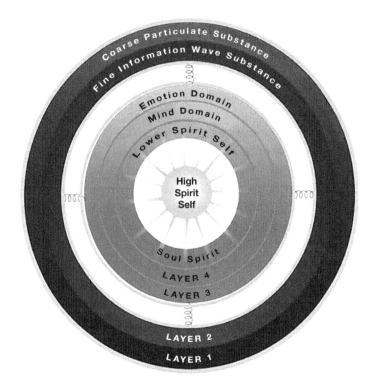

Figure 1. A metaphor for the whole person. I like to visualize a sphere composed of three concentric zones that are at least weakly coupled to each other. The outermost two layers are the personality self. The middle three layers are the soul self. The core region is the high-spirit self (or the God self).

At present, our global society thinks of *physical reality* as consisting of only one layer of substance, the electric atom/molecule layer of Figure 1. However, I prefer to define physical reality as consisting of the two layers of the personality self: the coarse, electric substance layer; and the fine, magnetic substance layer shown in Figure 1.

This second, inner layer of the personality self is where the acupuncture meridian system is thought to function. As many have experimentally discovered, there is no histological evidence of the acupuncture meridian system and its many acupuncture points that Dr. Shealy has highlighted in this book. At present, the only serious substantiation of this important structural system is of an electrodermal nature[2]. The acceptable evidence is a significantly enhanced electrical conductivity of the skin immediately

149

adjacent to the loci of the predicted locations of the acupuncture meridians and points.

When our souls are "born" into the space-time domain, the innermost magnetic substance layer (the old "etheric" layer) of our personality self is thought to form first and become the conventionally "invisible" template upon or around which the coarse, electric atom/molecule layer forms. All electrical-charge movement occurring in this outermost layer *induces* magnetic fields that are circulating around such electric current paths. These induced magnetic signatures are always of a dipolar nature rather than monopolar (see Figure 2)[3].

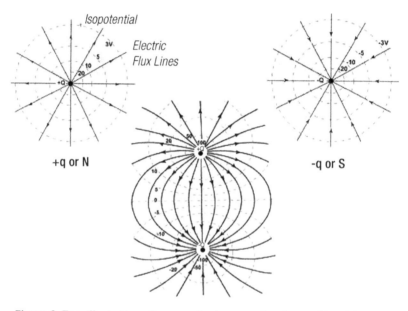

+q or N   -q or S

Figure 2. Top: illustration of monopoles (+q or –q for electric, N or S for magnetic); bottom: illustration of a dipole (+q –q for electric, NS for magnetic).

Thus, although we have experimentally isolated individual plus- and minus-signed electric charges and electric currents flowing in this outermost layer, only induced magnetic dipoles (N-S species) are present in this outermost layer.

Our experimental data[4-6] strongly suggests that magnetic monopoles and magnetic currents are present and functioning in this "invisible to electromagnetic sensors" template layer of the personality self.

Where Do These Electric Substances Come From?[7]

Paul Dirac (see endnote 7) was the first to meaningfully ask the question "Where do electrons come from?" He proposed that they were projected from the physical vacuum when a passing cosmic ray strongly *interacted with* the basic "stuff" of the physical vacuum (defined as having a complete absence of any electromagnetic matter, which does not mean empty). This cosmic-ray event was proposed to create an electron and its antimatter partner, the positron (see Figure 3).

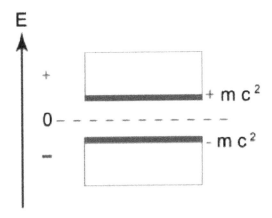

Figure 3. Schematic energy spectrum associated with the Dirac analysis. A band gap of forbidden energies exists between $E = \pm\, mc^2$ for particle-antiparticle creation of mass 2m.

This positron particle was eventually discovered by a subsequent experiment in the early 1930s, for which Dirac received a Nobel Prize.

Some years ago, I theoretically expanded Dirac's concept of Figure 3 to allow for the prevailing existence of additional layers of subtle energy substances (defined as: *all* substances *not* created via the four fundamental forces of today's orthodox science: gravity, electromagnetism [EM], the short-range nuclear force, and the long-range nuclear force). This working hypothesis is illustrated in Figure 4[8], with the soul self of Figure 1 being constructed from the three next higher-dimensional substances present in the physical vacuum (deeper in the physical vacuum than the magnetic information wave "stuff").

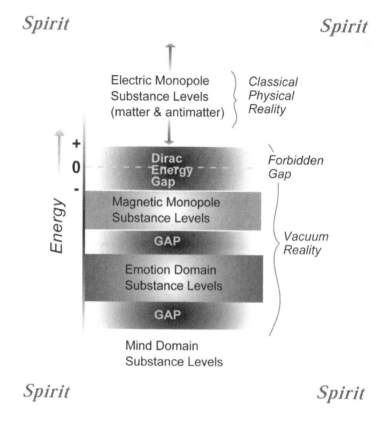

Figure 4. An energy-level diagram embracing both classical physical substances and "unseen" vacuum substances.

Thus, my working hypothesis is that the soul self is created from a composite of (1) emotion-domain materials, (2) mind-domain materials, and (3) some spirit-domain materials.

Experimentally, we have known for more than a century that, via both human sight and EM sensors, the physical vacuum is transparent to EM radiations of all frequencies, and that these photons travel at the same constant velocity, c, independent of the space-time distance through which they travel. Thus, these photons do not appear to significantly interact with any kind of "stuff" on their passage through physical vacuum.

This is the definition of a nondispersive medium, and it means that, for EM waves traveling through a physical vacuum, the EM wave velocity, v, is given by the simple formula:

$$V = \lambda \nu \quad (1)$$
Where λ = the wavelength and ν is the frequency of the EM wave.

Because of this simple formula, Eisberg[9] was able to show theoretically that, for the DeBroglie particle/pilotwave concept (experimentally confirmed in the 1920s) and the relativistic particle energy domain:

$$V_p = V_G \text{ and } V_p V_w = c^2. \quad (2)$$

(Here, V_p = particle velocity, V_w = pilotwave velocity,

and V_G = wave group velocity).

Thus, since V_p is less than c, always, V_w is greater than c, always, so it has a superluminal nature, and is therefore invisible to any EM sensor.

From the previous paragraph, my working hypothesis is that all the substance waves for those domains that lie deeper in the physical vacuum than V_w (the magnetic information wave) are also superluminal and thus transparent to our normal human eyesight and to today's orthodox science's EM sensors. This is why the human soul is not visible to today's orthodox science.

These insights, working hypotheses, and facts have been provided here because the five Shealy rings of Chapter Seven, and our future understanding of why they work so well to create such remarkable healing benefits for humans, are thought to depend upon this perspective.

References

1. W.A. Tiller, *Psychoenergetic Science: A Second Copernican-Scale Revolution* (Walnut Creek, CA: Pavior Publishing, 2007), 147–149.

2. W.A. Tiller, "On the Evolution and Future Development of Electrodermal Diagnostic Instruments" in *Energy Fields in Medicine*, ed. M.A. Morton and C. Dlouhy (Kalamazoo, MI: Fetzer Foundation, 1989).

3. Reference 1, p. 70, Figure 4.1.

4. Reference 1, p. 72, Figure 4.3.

5. W.A. Tiller; W.E. Dibble, Jr.; and M.J. Kohane, *Conscious Acts of Creation: The Emergence of a New Physics* (Walnut Creek, CA: Pavior Publishing, 2001).

6. W.A. Tiller; W.E. Dibble, Jr.; and J.G. Fandel, *Some Science Adventures with Real Magic* (Walnut Creek, CA: Pavior Publishing, 2005).

7. W.A. Tiller, "What Does the Dirac Negative Energy Sea Mean and Why Has Today's Orthodox Physics Neglected It?" online document, www.tiller.org, White Paper #VI.

8. Reference 1, pp. 154–155, Figure 7.7.

9. W.A. Tiller, "Why Has Orthodox Physics Neglected the Superluminal Velocities of the DeBroglie Pilot Wave Components?" online document, www.tiller.org, White Paper #V.

William A. Tiller, Ph.D.,

Emeritus Professor, Stanford University,

Department of Materials Science & Engineering

June 2013

BIBLIOGRAPHY

Akbar, N., Honarmand, K., and Feinstein, A. "Self-assessment of cognition in multiple sclerosis: the role of personality and anxiety." *Cognitive and Behavioral Neurology,* 24 (3) (2011): 115-21.

Armon, G. and Shirom, A. "The across-time associations of the five-factor model of personality with vigor and its facets using the bifactor model." *Journal of Personal Assessment,* 93 (6) (2011): 618-27.

Ayers, L.W., Missig, G., Schulkin, J., and Rosen, J.B. "Oxytocin reduces background anxiety in a fear-potentiated startle paradigm: peripheral vs. central administration." *Neuropsychopharmacology* (2011): 1-10.

Bales, K.L., Boone, E., Epperson, P., Hoffman, G., and Carter, C.S. "Are behavioral effects of early experience mediated by oxytocin?" *Frontiers in Psychiatry,* 2 (24) (2011).

Barraza, J.A., McCullough, M.E., Ahmadi, S., and Zak, P.J. "Oxytocin infusion increases charitable donations regardless of monetary resources." *Hormones and Behavior,* 60 (2011): 148-51.

Barrick, M., Mount, M., and Strauss, J. "Conscientiousness and performance of sales representatives: test of the mediating effects of goal setting." *Journal of Applied Psychology,* 78 (5) (1993): 715-722.

Bayles, A. *Eternal Triangle.* Madras, India: International Society for the Investigation of Ancient Civilizations (1988).

Breuil, V., Amri, E.Z., Panaia-Ferrari, P., Testa, J., Elabd, C., Albert-Sabonnadière, C., Roux, C.H., Ailhaud, G., Dani, C., Carle, G.F., and Euller-Ziegler, L. "Oxytocin and bone remodeling: relationships with neuropituitary hormones, bone status and body composition." *Joint, Bone, Spine* (2011). doi:10.1016.

Brooks, D. "Of Human Bonding." *New York Times* (July 2, 2006).

Bruce, J.M., Hancock, L.M., Arnett, P., and Lynch, S. "Treatment adherence in multiple sclerosis: association with emotional status, personality, and cognition." *Journal of Behavioral Medicine,* 33 (3) (2010): 219-27.

Bryant, R.A., Hung, L., Guastella, A.J., and Mitchell, P.B. "Oxytocin as a moderator of hypnotizability." *Psychoneuroendocrinology* (2011).

Buscaglia, L. *Love: What Life Is All About* . . . . New York: Fawcett Books (1972).

Cardoso, C., Ellenbogen, M.A., and Linnen, A.M. "Acute intranasal oxytocin improves positive self-perceptions of personality." *Psychopharmacology (Berl)*, 220 (4) (2012): 741-49.

Caska, C.M. and Renshaw, K.D. "Personality traits as moderators of the associations between deployment experiences and PTSD symptoms in OEF/OIF service members." *Anxiety, Stress, and Coping* (2011).

Chapman, B.P., van Wijngaarden, E., Seplaki, C.L., Talbot, N., Duberstein, P., and Moynihan, J. "Openness and conscientiousness predict 34-week patterns of interleukin-6 in older persons." *Brain, Behavior, and Immunity*, 25 (4) (2011): 667-73.

Chida, Y., Steptoe, A., and Powell, L.H. "Religiosity/spirituality and mortality. A systematic quantitative review." *Psychotherapy and Psychosomatics*, 78 (2) (2009): 81-90.

Colaianni, G., Di Benedetto, A., Zhu, L.L., Tamma, R., Li, J., Greco, G., Peng, Y., Dell'Endice, S., Zhu, G., Cuscito, C., Grano, M., Colucci, S., Iqbal, J., Yuen, T., Sun, L., Zaidi, M., and Zallones, A. "Regulated production of the pituitary hormone oxytocin from murine and human osteoblasts." *Biochemical and Biophysical Research Communications*, 411 (2011): 512-15.

Corker, K.S., Oswald, F.L., and Donnellan, M.B. "Conscientiousness in the classroom: a process explanation." *Journal of Personality* (2011).

Crocker, J., Luhtanen, R.K., Cooper, M.L., and Bouvrette, A. "Contingencies of self-worth in college students: theory and measurement." *Journal of Personality and Social Psychology*, 85 (5) (2003): 894-908.

De Dreu, C.K.W., Greer, L., Van Kleef, G., Shalvi, S., and Handgraaf, M. "Reply to Chen et al.: Perhaps goodwill is unlimited but oxytocin-induced goodwill is not." *PNAS*, 108 (13) (2011): E46.

Eaton, J.L., Roache, L., Nguyen, K.N., Cushing, B.S., Troyer, E., Papademetriou, E., and Raghanti, M.A. "Organizational effects of oxytocin on serotonin innervation." *Developmental Psychobiology* (April 2011).

Exton, N.G., Truong, T.C., Exton, M.S., Wingenfeld, S.A., Leygraf, N., Saller, B., Hartmann, U., and Schedlowski, M. "Neuroendocrine response to film-induced sexual arousal in men and women." *Psychoneuroendocrinology*, 25 (2000): 187-99.

Fallon, J., Avis, J., Kudisch, J., and Gornet, T. "Conscientiousness as a predictor of productive and counterproductive behaviors." *Journal of Business and Psychology*, 15 (2) (2000): 330-49.

Feldman, R., Gordon, I., and Zagoory-Sharon, O. "Maternal and paternal plasma, salivary, and urinary oxytocin and parent-infant synchrony: considering stress and affiliation components of human bonding." *Developmental Science*, 14 (4) (2011): 752-61.

Felitti, V. and Buczynski, R. "Why the most significant factor in predicting chronic disease may be childhood trauma." *National Institute for the Clinical Application of Behavioral Medicine* (September 13, 2011).

Freud, S. *On Creativity and the Unconscious: The Psychology of Art, Literature, Love, and Religion*. New York: Harper and Row (1958).

Friedman, H. and Martin, L. *The Longevity Project: Surprising Discoveries for Health and Long Life from the Landmark Eight-Decade Study*. New York: Penguin Group (2011).

Fromm, E. *The Art of Loving*. New York: Harper and Row (1956).

Grewen, K. and Light, K. "Plasma oxytocin is related to lower cardiovascular and sympathetic reactivity to stress." *Biological Psychology*, 87 (2011): 340.

Haber, J.R., Koenig, L.B., and Jacob, T. "Alcoholism, personality, and religion/spirituality: an integrative review." *Current Drug Abuse Reviews*, 4 (4) (2011): 250-60.

Hwang, J.Y., Shin, Y.C., Lim, S.W., Park, H.Y., Shin, N.Y., Jang, J.H., Park, H.Y., and Kwon, J.S. "Multidimensional comparison of personality characteristics of the big five model, impulsiveness, and affect in pathological gambling and obsessive-compulsive disorder." *Journal of Gambling Studies* (September 22, 2011).

Iverach, L., O'Brian, S., Jones, M., Block, S., Lincoln, M., Harrison, E., Hewat, S., Menzies, R.G., Packman, A., and Onslow, M. "The five factor model of personality applied to adults who stutter." *Journal of Communication Disorders*, 43 (2) (2010): 120-32.

Jackson, J., Balota, D.A., and Head, D. "Exploring the relationship between personality and regional brain volume in healthy aging." *Neurobiology of Aging*, 32 (12) (2011): 2162-71.

Janowski, K., Steuden, S., and Kurylowicz, J. "Factors accounting for psychosocial functioning in patients with low back pain." *European Spine Journal*, 19 (4) (2010): 613-23.

Jerant, A., Chapman, B., Duberstein, P., and Franks, P. "Effects of personality on self-rated health in a 1-year randomized controlled trial of chronic illness self-management." *British Journal of Health Psychology*, 15 (Pt2) (2010): 321-35.

Jones, M.P., Humphreys, J.S., and Nicholson, T. "Is personality the missing link in understanding recruitment and retention of rural general practitioners?" *Australian Journal of Rural Health*, 20 (2) (2012): 74-9.

Kern, M.L. and Friedman, H.S. "Do conscientious individuals live longer? A quantitative review." *Health Psychology*, 27 (5) (2008): 505-12.

Komisaruk, B.R. and Whipple, B. "Love as sensory stimulation: physiological consequences of its deprivation and expression." *Psychoneuroendocrinology*, 23 (8) (1998): 927-44.

Kurth, L. and Haussmann, R. "Perinatal Pitocin as an early ADHD biomarker: neurodevelopmental risk?" *Journal of Attention Disorders*, 15 (5) (2011): 423-431.

Leichtman, R. and Japikse, C. *Active Meditation: The Western Tradition.* Columbus, OH: Ariel Press (1982).

Lepine, J., Colquitt, J., and Erez, A. "Adaptability to changing task contexts: effects of general cognitive ability, conscientiousness, and openness to experience." *Personnel Psychology*, 53 (3) (2000): 563-93.

Levy, J.J. and Lounsbury, J.W. "Big five personality traits and performance anxiety in relation to marching arts satisfaction." *Work*, 40 (3) (2011): 297-302.

Lievens, F., Ones, D.S., and Dilchert, S. "Personality scale validities increase throughout medical school." *Journal of Applied Psychology*, 94 (6) (2009): 1514-35.

Lockenhoff, C.E., Duberstein, P.R., Friedman, B., and Costa, Jr., P.T. "Five-factor personality traits and subjective health among caregivers: the role of caregiver strain and self-efficacy." *Psychology and Aging*, 26 (3) (2011): 592-604.

Lukas, M., Toth, I., Reber, S., Slattery, D., Veenema, A., and Neumann, I. "The neuropeptide oxytocin facilitates pro-social behavior and prevents social avoidance in rats and mice." *Neuropsychopharmacology* (2011): 1-10.

MacLean, K., Johnson, M., and Griffiths, R. "Mystical experiences occasioned by the hallucinogen psilocybin lead to increases in the personality domain of openness." *Journal of Psychopharmacology*, 25 (11) (2008): 1453-61.

Maxson, P.J., Edwards, S.E., Ingram, A., and Miranda, M.L. "Psychosocial differences between smokers and non-smokers during pregnancy." *Addictive Behaviors*, 37 (2) (2012): 153-59.

Meyer-Luindenberg, A. "Impact of prosocial neuropeptides on human brain function." *Progress in Brain Research*, 170 (2008): 463-70.

Mitsui, S., Yamamoto, M., Nagasawa, M., Mogi, K., Kikusui, T., Ohtani, N., and Ohta, M. "Urinary oxytocin as a noninvasive biomarker of positive emotion in dogs." *Hormones and Behavior*, 60 (2011): 239-43.

Molnar, D.S., Sadava, S.W., Flett, G.L., and Colautti, J. "Perfectionism and health: a meditational analysis of the roles of stress, social support and health-related behaviors." *Psychology and Health* (2011).

Netherton, E. and Schatte, D. "Potential for oxytocin use in children and adolescents with mental illness." *Human Psychopharmacology*, 26 (2011): 271-81.

Norman, G.J., Hawkley, L.C., Cole, S.W., Berntson, G.G., and Cacioppo, J.T. "Social neuroscience: the social brain, oxytocin, and health." *Social Neuroscience*, (2011): 1-12.

Opacka-Juffry, J. and Mohiyeddini, C. "Experience of stress in childhood negatively correlates with plasma oxytocin concentration in adult men." *Stress*, 15 (1) (2011): 1-10. http://informahealthcare.com/doi/abs/10.310 9/10253890.2011.560309.

Pedersen, C.A. "Biological aspects of social bonding and the roots of human violence." *Annals of the New York Academy of Sciences*, 1036 (2004): 106-27.

Pedersen, C.A., Ascher, J.A., Monroe, Y.L., and Prange, Jr., A.J. "Oxytocin induces maternal behavior in virgin female rats." *Science*, 216 (4546) (1982): 648-50.

Power, C., Li, L., Atherton, K., and Hertzman, C. "Psychological health throughout life and adult cortisol patterns at age 45." *Psychoneuroendocrinology*, 36 (1) (2011): 87-97.

Riem, M.M., Bakermans-Kranenburg, M.J., Pieper, S., Tops, M., Boksem, M.A., Vermeiren, R.R., van Ijzendoorn, M.H., and Rombouts, S.A. "Oxytocin modulates amygdala, insula, and inferior frontal gyrus responses to infant crying: a randomized controlled trial." *Biological Psychiatry*, 70 (2011): 291-97.

Ring, R.H. "A complicated picture of oxytocin action in the central nervous system revealed." *Biological Psychiatry,* 69 (2011): 818-19.

Rise, M.B., Langvik, E., and Steinsbekk, A. "The personality of homeopaths: a cross-sectional survey of the personality profiles of homeopaths compared to a norm sample." *Journal of Alternative and Complementary Medicine,* 18 (1) (2012): 42-47.

Rockliff, H., Karl, A., McEwan, K., Gilbert, J., Matos, M., and Gilbert, P. "Effects of intranasal oxytocin on 'compassion focused imagery.'" *Emotion* (2011).

Ryman, S., Gasparovic, C., Bedrick, E., Flores, R., Marshall, A., and Jung, R. "Brain biochemistry and personality: a magnetic resonance spectroscopy study." (November 3, 2011). www.plosone.org/article/info%3A doi%2F10.1371%2Fjournal.pone.0026758

Sackett, P. and Wanek, J. "New developments in the use of measures of honesty, integrity, conscientiousness, dependability, trustworthiness, and reliability for personnel selection." *Personnel Psychology,* 49 (4) (1996): 787-829.

Saraydarian, T. *Irritation: The Destructive Fire.* Cave Creek, AZ: Publishing Foundation (1991).

Scantamburlo, G., Ansseau, M., Geenen, V., and Legros, J.J. "Oxytocin: from milk ejection to maladaptation in stress response and psychiatric disorders. A psychoneuroendocrine perspective." *Annales d'Endocrinologie,* 70 (2009): 449-54.

Scantamburlo, G., Ansseau, M., Geenen, V., and Legros, J.J. *Journal of Neuropsychiatry and Clinical Neurosciences,* (2011): 23, 2.

Schulze, L., Lischke, A., Greif, J., Herpertz, S.C., Heinrichs, M., and Domes, G. "Oxytocin increases recognition of masked emotional faces." *Psychoneuroendocrinology,* 36 (9) (October 2011): 1378-82.

Sikrundz, M., Bolten, M., Nast, I., Hellhammer, D., and Meinlschmidt, G. "Plasma oxytocin concentration during pregnancy is associated with development of postpartum depression." *Neuropsychopharmacology,* 36 (2011): 1886-93.

Simeon, D., Bartz, J., Hamilton, H., Crystal, S., Braun, A., Ketay, S., and Hollander, E. "Oxytocin administration attenuates stress reactivity in borderline personality disorder: a pilot study." *Psychoneuroendocrinology* (2011).

Sipiora, M. "Obligations Beyond Competency: Metabletics as a Conscientious Psychology." *Janus Head,* 10 (2) (2008): 425-43.

Slattery, D. and Neumann, D. "Oxytocin and major depressive disorder: experimental and clinical evidence for links to aetiology and possible treatment." *Pharmaceuticals,* 3 (2010): 702-24.

Smith, T.W. and MacKenzie, J. "Personality and risk of physical illness." *Annual Review of Clinical Psychology,* 2 (2006): 435-67.

Specht, J., Egloff, B., and Schmukle, S.C. "Stability and change of personality across the life course: the impact of age and major life events on mean-level and rank-order stability of the Big Five." *Journal of Personal and Social Psychology,* 101 (4) (2011): 862-82.

Steinhausen, H.C., Göllner, J., Brandeis, D., Müller, U.C., Valko, L., and Drechsler, R. "Psychopathology and personality in parents of children with ADHD." *Journal of Attention Disorders* (March 5, 2012).

Striepens, N., Kendrick, K.M., Maier, W., and Hurlemann, R. "Prosocial effects of oxytocin and clinical evidence for its therapeutic potential." *Frontiers in Neuroendocrinology* (July 1, 2011).

Tackett, J., Slobodskaya, H., Mar, R., Deal, J., Halverson, Jr., C., Baker, S., Pavlopoulos, V., and Besevegis, E. "The hierarchical structure of childhood personality in five countries: continuity from early childhood to early adolescence." *Journal of Personality* (2011).

Takahashi, Y., Roberts, B.W., and Hoshino, T. "Conscientiousness mediates the relation between perceived parental socialization and self-rated health." *Psychology & Health,* 20 (2) (2012): 74-79.

The Readings Research Department and Cayce, E. *Attitudes and Emotions: Part II (The Edgar Cayce Readings Vol. 14).* Virginia Beach: Association of Research and Enlightenment, Inc. xiv (1982): 767.

Timmer, M., Cordero, M.I., Sevelinges, Y., and Sandi, C. "Evidence for a role of oxytocin receptors in the long-term establishment of dominance hierarchies." *Neuropsychopharmacology* (2011): 108.

Tolea, M.I., Costa, Jr., P.T., Terracciano, A., Ferrucci, L., Faulkner, K., Coday, M.M., Ayonayon, H.N., and Simonsick, E.M. "Associations of openness and conscientiousness with walking speed decline: findings from the health, aging, and body composition study." *Journals of Gerontology. Series B, Psychological Sciences and Social Sciences* (March 26, 2012).

Turiano, N.A., Pitzer, L., Armour, C., Karlamangla, A., Ryff, C.D., and Mroczek, D.K. "Personality trait level and change as predictors of health outcomes: findings from a national study of Americans (MIDUS)." *Journals of Gerontology. Series B, Psychological Sciences and Social Sciences,* 67B (1) (July 15, 2011): 4-12.

Umaki, T.M., Umaki, M.R., and Cobb, C.M. "The psychology of patient compliance: a focused review of the literature." *Journal of Periodontology,* 83 (4) (2012): 395-400.

Van Anders, S.M., Goldey, K.L., and Kuo, P.X. "The steroid/peptide theory of social bonds: integrating testosterone and peptide responses for classifying social behavioral contexts." *Psychoneuroendocrinology* (2011).

Van den Hurk, P., Wingens, T., Giommi, F., Barendregt, H., Speckens, A., and van Schie, T. "On the relationship between the practice of mindfulness meditation and personality—an exploratory analysis of the mediating role of mindfulness skills." *Mindfulness,* 2 (3) (2011): 194-200.

Weber, K., Giannakopoulos, P., Bacchetta, J.P., Quast, S., Hermann, F.R., Delaloye, C., Ghisletta, P., De Ribaupierre, A., and Canuto, A. "Personality traits are associated with acute major depression across the age spectrum." *Aging & Mental Health* (2011).

Weisbuch, M., Ambady, N., Slepian, M.L., and Jimerson, D.C. "Emotion contagion moderates the relationship between emotionally-negative families and abnormal eating behavior." *International Journal of Eating Disorders,* 44 (8) (2011): 716-20.

Weiss, A., Sutin, A.R., Duberstein, P.R., Friedman, B., Bagby, R.M., and Costa, Jr., P.T. "The personality domains and styles of the five-factor model are related to incident depression in Medicare recipients aged 65 to 100." *American Journal of Geriatric Psychiatry,* 17 (7) (2009): 591-601.

Welch, H.G. "If You Feel O.K., Maybe You Are O.K." *New York Times* (February 27, 2012).

Wresinska, M.A. and Kocur, J. "The assessment of personality traits and coping style level among the patients with functional dyspepsia and irritable bowel syndrome." *Psychiatria Polska,* 42 (5) (2008): 709-17.

Ystrom, E., Vollrath, M.E., and Nordeng, H. "Effects of personality on use of medications, alcohol, and cigarettes during pregnancy." *European Journal of Clinical Pharmacology* (December 22, 2011).

Zeleznik, U. "The physician between the ideal and reality: medical profession and popular attitude towards health and medicine in the 19th century." *Acta Medico-Historica Adriatica,* 8 (2) (2010): 293-328.

᠅ ᠅ ᠅ ᠅ ᠅ ᠅

ACKNOWLEDGMENTS

I appreciate the fact that I have taken the road *less traveled;* it was the most conscientious route I could find! I choose to continue this path as long as I can take care of myself and provide some help to others. I believe, first and foremost, that I must first do good for myself in order to have the energy to do good for others. I am pleased to acknowledge the people here who have made the most delightful difference in my life.

My Family: My mother; father; sisters Mary and Linda; Grandmother Padget; Great-Grandmother Rickard; Great-Great-Grandfather Smith; Aunt Louise; Aunt Dorothy; Aunt Frances; Great-Aunt Eva; Great-Uncle Tommy; Uncles Lever, B.N., Brinton, and Freeman; cousins Lillian, Ellen, Frank, and Roy; a score of second and third cousins; and of course my wife, Mary-Charlotte; our children, Brock, Craig, and Laurel, and their spouses, plus our grandchildren, Sophia, Jared, Natalie, Lexi, and Joshua. For more than 52 years, Mary-Charlotte provided me the solid support and nurturing that allowed me to develop all the tools that I found to assist others in achieving greater heath.

Extraordinary Teachers: Miss Ada; Miss Taylor; Willie Tiller; Mrs. Funderburke; James Sheeley; Talmage Peele; Eugene A. Stead, Jr.; Jack Myers; Henry McIntosh; Carl Moyer; Frank Engle; Herb Lourie; Tom Ballantine; Sam Keen; Jack Schwartz; Bella Karrasch; Elmer Green; Henry Rucker; Bob Leichtman; Caroline Myss; Deena Spear; Marianne Alexander; Cay Randall-May; Bill Farber; and scores of others.

Friends: Several hundred, but with very special thanks to Robert, Mutt, Jim, Rick, Harry, Ed, Gordon, Gladys, Roger, Joe, Bill, Joe, Bob, Ann, Fred, Caroline, Robert, Julie, and Lucia.

Editorial and Publishing: I am grateful to the team at Hay House for their valuable assistance in the production and promotion of this book. I am indebted to my staff members in Missouri who help me keep the farm and our companies so well organized and running smoothly. And I appreciate the help of my conscientious editor and advisor on this project, Simone Graham, who worked with me to get this manuscript ready for publication.

◡◡◡ ◡◡◡

ABOUT THE AUTHOR

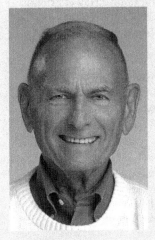

C. Norman Shealy MD, PhD is one of the world's leading experts in pain management. He was the first physician to specialize in the resolution of chronic pain, and his intensive research into pain and stress management led to the pioneering of more than a dozen safe and effective treatments, therapies and patents – including Biogenics. In 1971, Dr Shealy founded the first comprehensive pain- and stress-management facility in the USA, namely The Shealy Institute, respected worldwide for its innovative and successful rehabilitation approaches.

His seminars and workshops are given worldwide, and are attended by physicians and laypersons alike. His published works total over 325, including 29 books. Dr Shealy is Senior Fellow Emeritus with the Biofeedback Certification Institute of America as of 2003, and he was granted the O. Spurgeon English Humanitarian Award for 2002 by Temple University. He also cofounded the American Board for Scientific Medical Intuition (ABSMI), is a Professor Emeritus of Energy Medicine with Greenwich University and was named a founding diplomate of the American Board of Holistic Medicine in 2000.

www.normshealy.com

Hay House Titles of Related Interest

YOU CAN HEAL YOUR LIFE, the movie, starring Louise Hay & Friends
(available as a 1-DVD programme and an expanded 2-DVD set)
Watch the trailer at: www.LouiseHayMovie.com

THE SHIFT, the movie,
starring Dr Wayne W. Dyer
(available as a 1-DVD program and an expanded 2-DVD set)
Watch the trailer at: www.DyerMovie.com

❧ ❧ ❧

DEFY GRAVITY: Healing Beyond the Bounds of Reason, by Caroline Myss

INSIDE-OUT HEALING: Transforming Your Life Through the Power of Presence, by Richard Moss

THE MAN WHO DROVE WITH HIS EYES CLOSED,
by The Barefoot Doctor

OUR RETURN TO THE LIGHT: A New Path to Health and Healing,
by Barbara Wren

SIMPLY GENIUS! And Other Tales from My Life, by Ervin Laszlo

STOP PAIN: Inflammation Relief for an Active Life, by Vijay Vad MD

All of the above are available at your local bookstore,
or may be ordered by contacting Hay House (see next page).

❧ ❧ ❧

We hope you enjoyed this Hay House book. If you'd like to receive our online catalogue featuring additional information on Hay House books and products, or if you'd like to find out more about the Hay Foundation, please contact:

Hay House UK, Ltd.,
Astley House, 33 Notting Hill Gate, London W11 3JQ
Phone: 0-20-3675-2450 • *Fax:* 0-20-3675-2451
www.hayhouse.co.uk • www.hayfoundation.org

ᴗ ᴗ

Published and distributed in the United States by:
Hay House, Inc., P.O. Box 5100, Carlsbad, CA 92018-5100
Phone: (760) 431-7695 or (800) 654-5126
Fax: (760) 431-6948 or (800) 650-5115
www.hayhouse.com®

Published and distributed in Australia by:
Hay House Australia Pty. Ltd., 18/36 Ralph St., Alexandria NSW 2015
Phone: 612-9669-4299 • *Fax:* 612-9669-4144 • www.hayhouse.com.au

Published and distributed in the Republic of South Africa by:
Hay House SA (Pty), Ltd., P.O. Box 990, Witkoppen 2068
Phone/Fax: 27-11-467-8904 • www.hayhouse.co.za

Published in India by:
Hay House Publishers India, Muskaan Complex,
Plot No. 3, B-2, Vasant Kunj, New Delhi 110 070
Phone: 91-11-4176-1620 • *Fax:* 91-11-4176-1630 • www.hayhouse.co.in

Distributed in Canada by:
Raincoast Books, 2440 Viking Way, Richmond, B.C. V6V 1N2
Phone: 1-800-663-5714 • *Fax:* 1-800-565-3770 • www.raincoast.com

ᴗ ᴗ ᴗ

Take Your Soul on a Vacation

Visit www.HealYourLife.com® to regroup,
recharge, and reconnect with your own magnificence.
Featuring blogs, mind-body-spirit news, and
life-changing wisdom from Louise Hay and friends.

Visit www.HealYourLife.com today

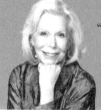
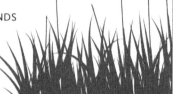